ExAM for Critical Care

Charles F. Swearingen

ISBN: 1533462593
ISBN-13: 978-1533462596

DEDICATION

This book I dedicate to the critical care student. To master critical care as a non-physician, you need to understand that you'll never actually master it. It will always teach you that you'll need to study a little more. That being said, my message isn't to avoid studying the fascinating topics within the critical care realm, rather we need to harness other clinicians knowledge by reading, practicing, asking questions, and leaning as much as we can. If we do this, then we can approach our clinician potentials and best take care of our patients. So, I raise a metaphorical glass to you, the critical care student who charges ahead in our field of transport medicine. You are our champions of tomorrow. Thank you for the good fight.

CONTENTS

ACKNOWLEDGMENTS

With this text, I sent a call out for peer reviewers to identify errors in this manuscript. Over 100 people responded to which I put to work. Thank all of you for being willing to undertake such an endeavor and thank you for continuing to strive to be the best clinician you can. I am honored so many of you answered the call. Below are all the individuals who helped to review this textbook.

1 TRAUMA

Questions

1. Your trauma patient has suffered massive bleeding. Which of the following treatments would improve perfusion the most?

   A. Packed RBCs
   B. Fluids wide open
   C. Vasopressors
   D. Anticoagulants

2. Your trauma patient presents with difficulty breathing. The patient's vitals are as follows HR 109, BP 90/62 (producing a weak radial pulse), and percussion produces a dull chest sensation. What is the patient's current condition?

   A. Tamponade
   B. Pnnumothorax
   C. Hemothorax
   D. Flail Segment

3. You notice dark red blood oozing from a 2 cm laceration from your patient's right hand. What is the most appropriate management for this patient?

   A. Ventilation
   B. Keep warm
   C. Direct pressure
   D. Tourniquet

4. Your patient's HCT is 19%. What is the best treatment for this situation?

   A. Blood Products
   B. Isotonic Crystalloids
   C. Lactated Ringers
   D. Hypertonic Saline

5. Your trauma patient just experienced a head on collision with another vehicle. Their injuries include pulmonary contusions, burns forearms, and bilateral broken femurs. What injury patterns are they displaying?

   A. Laying the bike down
   B. Down and Under
   C. Up and Over Pathway
   D. Lateral Impact

6. A patient in your care is hypotensive from injuries from a MVC. Currently, their HGB is 6.8 g/dL. Interpret this finding.

   A. Critical High
   B. Critical Low
   C. Normal
   D. High
   E. Low

7. Your GSW patient has an entrance wound at their forehead, and a large hole at their occipitut. This was caused by a single gunshot. What can you infer from this information?

   A. It was low velocity a long distance away
   B. It was high velocity and at closer range.
   C. It was low velocity at a nearby distance
   D. It was high velocity a long distance away

8. Your patient has been involved in an MVC. The patient presents with a fractured nose, fractures to both thighs, and JVD following impacting another vehicle head- on. What injury patterns are they displaying?

   A. Lateral Impact
   B. Down and Under
   C. Laying the bike down
   D. Up and Over Pathway

9. Your MVC patient wrecked their vehicle due to an over dose of benzodiazepines. As you arrive, the patient is noted to be bradypneic (3 breaths/min). You have an open airway. What is the most appropriate management strategy?

   A. Ventilation
   B. Suction
   C. Intubation
   D. Reposition

10. A patient is involved in a frontal impact MVC. The patient presents with fractured lower leg bones on both sides, severe hip crepitus, and fractured patellas. What injury patterns are they displaying?

   A. Down and Under Pathway
   B. Up and Over Pathway
   C. Laying the bike down
   D. Lateral Impact

11. A trauma patient you are assessing just experienced a MVC. They are not following commands and are grabbing your wrists throughout the exam. They look at you directly, yet talks in sounds that are not words. In which step do they meet trauma criteria?

   A. Step 1
   B. Step 2
   C. Step 3
   D. Step 4

12. Your patient was in a house fire 24 hours ago and suffered 19% partial thickness burns. You note a HGB 23 g/dL. Interpret this finding.

    A. Critical High
    B. Critical Low
    C. Normal
    D. High

13. A patient presents with a stab wound to the left upper quadrant. Which of the following would most significantly indicate peritoneal hemorrhage?

    A. Back pain
    B. High EtCO2
    C. Pale skin
    D. Hypertension

14. Your patient has been crushed by a pile of dirt that fell out of a bulldozer's scoop and onto the patient. Rescuers have cleared his head from dirt. What should the critical care clinician be considering at this point?

    A. Perform needle decompression
    B. Begin a buffering infusion right away
    C. Initiate IV fluids before he is freed
    D. Prepare for intubation once he is free

15. You have a patient that presents with the following vital signs and findings: HR 102, BP 94/65, RR24, (+) left shoulder pain and Grey- Turner's sign. Which of the following conditions does this most suggest?

    A. Splenic Injury
    B. Liver Injury
    C. Great Vessel Injury
    D. Intestinal Injury

16. Your trauma patient is exhibiting left sided paresthesia and hemiparesis. He also is not alert to time or place. With this information you know that the patient meets criteria for which hospital?

    A. Level I
    B. Level II
    C. Level III
    D. Level IV

17. Upon exposing a female patient who was involved in a 2 story fall, you note a large laceration on the pubic mound. What is the most appropriate initial management for this patient?

    A. Begin BVM ventilations
    B. Start 2 Large bore IVs
    C. Apply a pelvic binder
    D. Apply a traction splint

18. A patient has been assaulted with a baseball bat to the head and neck. You note bubbling in the airway with each respiration. What is the most appropriate management strategy?

    A. Reposition
    B. Intubation
    C. Suction
    D. Ventilation

19. You have a patient that presents with the following vital signs and findings: HR 120, BP 82/55, RR24, (+) seatbelt sign, rebound tenderness, and vomiting. Which of the following conditions does this most suggest?

    A. Splenic Injury
    B. Liver Injury
    C. Great Vessel Injury
    D. Intestinal Injury

20. You administer 3 unit of PRBCs to your hypotensive trauma patient. What should their HCT elevate to if it was 36% before being administered blood?

    A. 39%
    B. 41%
    C. 43%
    D. 45%

21. After examining the labs of your trauma patient, you note longer than normal clotting times. Which of the following medications should you administer?

    A. Heparin
    B. Vitamin K
    C. Warfarin
    D. Cryoprecip

22. You're transporting a patient from a smaller hospital to a larger regional hospital for multisystem trauma care. The patient is on an IV antibiotic. The astute critical care transport clinician will be monitoring for systemic effects. Which of the following represents a systemic allergic reaction (anaphylaxis)?

    A. Uticaria and wheezing
    B. Severe hypotension
    C. Tall peaked T- waves
    D. Small dull U- waves

23. Your patient suffered a serious head laceration and lost a significant amount of blood. Their hematocrit is 11%. Interpret this finding.

    A. Critical High
    B. Critical Low
    C. Normal
    D. High
    E. Low

24. You administer 500 cc of PRBCs to your hypotensive trauma patient. What should their Hgb elevate to if the Hgb was 10 g/dL before being administered blood?

    A. 14 g/dL
    B. 12 g/dL
    C. 16 g/dL
    D. 18 g/dL

25. Your GI bleed patient is hypotensive. Their hematocrit is 23%. Interpret this finding.

    A. Critical High
    B. Critical Low
    C. Normal
    D. High
    E. Low

26. Consider the following items. Pick the one which would cause the greatest tissue crush.

    A. Steak knife
    B. A pick axe
    C. Baseball bat
    D. Pair of scissors

27. Upon assessment, your trauma patient is found to have an open book pelvis and severe pain during the pelvic rock. With this information you know that the patient meets criteria for which hospital?

A. Level I
B. Level II
C. Level III
D. Level IV

28. You have a patient who suffered blunt force trauma. At the sending facility, the patient presented with extreme shortness of breath, 120/78 BP, SpO2 of 93% and is being treated appropriately with ABCs, CPAP with 10-15 PEEP, fluids and pain meds. What do you suggest the underlying pathophysiology is?

A. Intestinal Contusion
B. Pulmonary Contusion
C. Cardiac Tamponade
D. Pericardial Effusion

29. A patient involved in an explosion and has a 3 cm opening in his chest that has been covered with an occlusive dressing tapped on 3 sides. The patient vital signs: HR 110, BP 80/50, pulse ox 82%. What is the most appropriate treatment?

A. Burp the chest dressing
B. Decompress the chest
C. Remove chest dressing
D. Tape the 4th side down

30. A patient who was the victim of an assault has suffered peritoneal bleeding. Which of the following findings indicates the pathology is blood collecting at the diaphragm?

    A. Kehr's Sign
    B. Bruzinski's Sign
    C. Cullen's Sign
    D. Beck's Sign

31. What is the lab profile for a rhabdomyolysis patient?

    A. High K, Low Ca, norm H/H
    B. Low H/H, high K, normal Ca
    C. Normal K, high Ca, normal H/H
    D. Low K, Low Ca, normal H/H

32. You examine a patient who was a victim in a massive 15 car pileup. The patient presents with deep abrasions to his left leg, left arm and left torso. Additionally, he has a left ulnar fracture. What injury patterns are they displaying?

    A. Up and Over Pathway
    B. Laying the bike down
    C. Down and Under
    D. Lateral Impact

33. You administer 3 units of PRBCs to your hypotensive trauma patient. What should their HGB elevate to if the HGB was 7 g/dL before being administered blood?

A. 8 g/dL
B. 9 g/dL
C. 10 g/dL
D. 11 g/dL

34. Your trauma patient has experienced significant blood loss. The ER staff report the lactate to be 6 mmol/L after administering 1000cc NS and 2 units of PRBCs 60 minutes prior. You are transporting this patient to a Level I hospital. Was the hospital's treatment effective?

A. **YES**. They have almost replaced the volume lost and the patient is most likely stabilized.
B. **NO**. The lactate is critically high. They have only given 1250 cc of fluid (1000 NS and 250cc of PRBCs). The patient needs more fluid and PRBCs.
C. **YES**. This lactate value matches the normal range of oxygen saturation in the venous system.
D. **NEED MORE INFORMATION**.

35. Following an MVC (car vs. pedestrian), your patient presents with a shortened left leg with crepitus and deformation. There is currently no pulse distal the deformity. What is the best initial management for this patient?

A. Splint the extremity as is
B. Reposition without traction
C. Traction and reposition
D. Put in closed packed position

36. A patient experiences a frontal impact MVC. Which of the following is consistent with the 'down and under' injury pattern?

A. Fractured patellas
B. Bi-lateral Femur fxs
C. Scaphoid fracture
D. Transverse process fx

37. Your trauma patient currently has 2 chest tubes that are collecting blood at a rapid rate. You decide it best to administer 2 units of O negative blood. What would you anticipate the HCT to be an hour later if the original HCT was 17%?

A. 20%
B. 23%
C. 18%
D. 25%

38. The sending facility has administered protamine sulfate to your trauma patient. Which of the following conditions do you suspect in your patients?

A. Low H/H
B. High Crit
C. Low PT
D. High PTT

39. Your pregnant patient presents with Kehr's sign and hypotension. What injury are they most likely experiencing?

    A. Uterine Rupture
    B. Intestinal Injury
    C. Splenic Injury
    D. Abruptio Placenta

40. Upon assessing your patient who just suffered an MVC, you note an abrasion to the forehead, inappropriate responses to simple answers and a blood pressure of 72/50. Distal pulses are absent. With this information you know that the patient meets criteria for which hospital?

    A. Level I
    B. Level II
    C. Level III
    D. Level IV

41. Upon assessment, your patient presents from an MVC with severe shortness of breath, severe air hunger, massive subcutaneous air in the in the anterior chest, and equal, clear, but faint breath sounds. What condition is most likely the reason for these symptoms?

    A. Tension pneumothorax
    B. Pulmonary contusion
    C. Pericardial Effusion
    D. Tracheobronchial injury

42. Your patient has experienced a rollover MVC and presents with right upper quadrant pain, pale skin, and diffuse right shoulder pain. What is the patient most likely suffering from?

    A. Intestinal Injury
    B. Liver Injury
    C. Splenic Injury
    D. Diaphragmatic Injury

43. You administer 500 cc of PRBCs to your hypotensive trauma patient. What should their HCT elevate to if it was 19% before being administered blood?

    A. 25%
    B. 29%
    C. 31%
    D. 33%

44. Your patient has been assaulted with a crowbar and was struck multiple times in the chest with it. They present with asymmetrical chest wall with each inspiration but there is no paradoxical motion. What is the most appropriate management for this patient?

    A. Immediate ventilation
    B. Needle decompression
    C. Reposition the airway
    D. Splint with bulky pad

45. You have an adult patient who is exhibiting deep respirations and who doesn't answer when you call out to him. He has dry, rattling breath sounds. What is the most appropriate management strategy?

    A. Suction
    B. Ventilation
    C. Intubation
    D. Reposition

46. A painter fell off of a 2 story house and landed on hard dirt impacting his feet. The patient presents as follows: HR 101 BP 98/59 RR 14, (+) pulses with a shortened right leg, and is awake and alert. No other injuries are present. What treatment MUST occur?

    A. Hip binding with sheet
    B. Begin bilateral large IVs
    C. Administer pain meds
    D. Initiate NS fluid bolus

47. Your patient has experienced significant abdominal trauma. Their current vitals are HR 108, RR 29, mottled skin, and delayed capillary refill. What is the most appropriate management for this patient?

    A. Obtain an H and H
    B. Administer fluid bolus
    C. Administer pressors
    D. Put in Trendelenburg

48. You're transporting a patient from a smaller hospital to a larger regional hospital for multisystem trauma care. The patient is on an IV antibiotic. The astute critical care transport clinician understands which of the following to be a mild to moderate allergic reaction?

A. Uticaria and wheezing
B. Severe hypotension
C. Tall peaked T- waves
D. Small dull U- waves

49. Your patient has attempted suicide by slicing their wrist and they lost approximately 1.5 L of blood. They have a HGB of 4.9 g/dL. Interpret these findings.

A. Critical High
B. Critical Low
C. Normal
D. High
E. Low

50. A bicyclist was struck at 25 MPH crossing a busy intersection and then run over by a second vehicle. He states he is just sore and would rather go home to rest. If you convinced him to go to the hospital, in which step do they meet trauma criteria?

A. Step 1
B. Step 2
C. Step 3
D. Step 4

51. Upon assessing your trauma patient, you note calcaneus and scaphoid fractures bilaterally as well as an acetabular fracture. What injury pattern is being displayed here?

A. Rotational Impact
B. Up and Over
C. Down and Under
D. Critical Fall

52. You are assessing a patient who suffered a MVC as the restrained driver. You note crepitus to left hip and left femur as well as notice shattered glass in their hair on their left side. What injury pattern is being displayed here?

A. Down and Under Pathway
B. Up and Over Pathway
C. Laying the bike down
D. Lateral Impact

53. Your trauma patient impacted the steering wheel during a frontal impact MVC. There is crepitus over the rib just inferior to the left clavicle with ecchymosis and there is a 16 mmHg difference between the right and left arm. What condition is the patient experiencing?

A. Flail segment
B. Pulmonary contusion
C. Aortic rupture
D. Cardiac contusion

54. Your patient received blunt force trauma to their leg. The patient presents as follows: HR 103, BP 118/78, RR 19, (+) weak pulse to RLE, moves all extremities, and is awake and alert. No other injuries are present. What condition is most likely present?

A. Femur fracture present
B. Pelvic fracture present
C. Rhabdomyolysis
D. Compartment syndrome

55. A young adult has received a steering wheel impact in a MVC. He has no medical problems, but now is presenting with shortness of breath and fine rales are present. You intubate the patient. What ventilator settings would most likely be appropriate?

A. Applying PEEP at 11 cmH2O
B. RR matching minute ventilation
C. I:E allowing for reduced exhalation
D. Minimize FiO2 preventing hyperoxia

56. You note a SvO2 of 62% on your trauma patient's lab panel. What is the best treatment for this?

A. Hypertonic Saline
B. Blood plasma
C. Isotonic Crystalloids
D. Lactated Ringers

57. Your MVC patient has some minor injuries and answers questions appropriately. There was a death in the same vehicle and minimal damage to the patient's vehicle. In which step do they meet trauma criteria?

A. Step 1
B. Step 2
C. Step 3
D. Step 4

58. An adult gets his foot caught in a farming combine, and severs half of his foot off. How would you field triage this patient?

A. Closest appropriate
B. Teaching hospital
C. County hospital
D. Level 1 Trauma

59. A patient has been involved in an assault with a baseball bat and was struck several times to the lower half of his body. He has pelvic fractures and hypotension. His vitals are BP 80/68, HR 108, SpO2 95%. How should you best treat this patient?

A. Administer fluids
B. Insert a Foley cath
C. Begin Dopamine
D. Permissive hypotension

60. Your patient has suffered a stabbing to the chest at the 5th intercostal space 3 inches to the left of their midline. He is exhibiting breathing difficulty, a weak pulse, and CVP of 16 and wedge pressure of 23. Which condition are you suspecting?

A. Cardiac rupture
B. Tension pneumothorax
C. Massive hemothorax
D. Cardiac tamponade

61. Your young adult trauma patient was thrown from a motorcycle and impacted the pavement. He is exhibiting ST elevation in leads II, III, and aVF with a wide QRS in V1. What condition is the patient most likely experiencing?

A. Cardiac Contusion
B. Cardiac Tamponade
C. Pericardial Effusion
D. Pulmonary contusion

62. Upon responding to an MVC, you assess your patient to discover significant crepitus to the occipital region. With this injury there is an indention to the occipital region itself. With this information you know that the patient meets criteria for which hospital?

A. Teaching hospital
B. Closest appropriate
C. Level 1 Trauma
D. County hospital

63. The sending facility has administered anticoagulants to your trauma patient. Which of the following conditions do you suspect in your patients?

A. PID
B. CAD
C. DIC
D. CHF

64. Enroute to the hospital which a multitrauma MVC patient, your ventilator sounds the high pressure alarm. Upon assessment, you notice unsymmetrical chest rise and fall and JVD. What is the most appropriate management for this patient?

A. Ventilate with BVM
B. Needle decompress
C. Re-intubate the patient
D. Check plateau pressure

65. If you administer 750 cc of PRBCs to a patient, and their hemoglobin changes from 9 g/dL to 11 g/dL, then what do you suspect is happening?

A. Normal HGB finding
B. Appropriate response
C. Hemorrhage continues
D. Hypercoagulation

66. A colleague is explaining that a football player had been recently transported for rhabdomyolysis. You know that this condition is best treated by which of the following:

    A. Normal saline, potassium
    B. Fluids, bicarb, calcium
    C. Potassium, bicarb, fluids
    D. Fluids, analgesics, B- blocker

67. Your patient was struck by a vehicle impacting his chest and head. Currently, their vitals are: HR 118, pulse ox 82%, BP 88/52 (bilaterally). You observe absent breath sounds on the right side and on the left exists a hyporesonant chest. What do you suspect is the condition?

    A. Aortic rupture
    B. Pneumothorax
    C. Hemothorax
    D. Flail segment

68. A patient has been stabbed with a wide knife that is approximately 8 inches long. The wound is to the right of midline on the abdomen approximately 3 inches above the level of the umbilicus. Reportedly, the stabbing motion was upward. The patient vital signs: HR 112, RR 27, pulse ox 88%, BP 122/80, GCS of 15. What is the most appropriate treatment of this patient?

    A. Place a chest tube
    B. Insert an ET tube
    C. Needle decompression
    D. Give BVM ventilations

69. Your pregnant patient has suffered direct blunt trauma to her abdomen and is concerned that her unborn child is injured or in danger. Which of the following would most indicate danger to the fetus?

 A. Left shoulder pain
 B. Right shoulder pain
 C. Intense nausea
 D. Sharp back pain

70. A trauma patient in your care has a lactate of 3.2. What is the best treatment for this patient?

 A. Reduce CO2
 B. Pain meds
 C. Increase RR
 D. Restore BP

71. Your young adult trauma patient has been in a significant rollover MVC. Upon auscultation, you cannot hear heart tones, the patient has a weak carotid pulse, (JVD), and clear lung sounds. What immediate treatment is warranted?

 A. Withdraw pericardial fluid
 B. Remove air from the pleura
 C. Increase the tidal volume
 D. Reduce PEEP on the vent

72. An explosive device lifts a car next to it upon detonation and throws it into a nearby crowd. Three (3) people are struck and injured by the car. What injury pattern is exhibited here?

    A. Primary blast
    B. Secondary blast
    C. Tertiary blast
    D. Quaternary blast

Answers

1. (**A**) PRBCs is the only thing that will increase the oxygen carrying capacity of the blood, and thus the only thing that will improve perfusion.

2. (**C**) The dull lung sound in this question points to the way a chest feels when it is filled with fluid. You won't get that feeling, or sensation, with these other conditions.

3. (**C**) Even though this is a venous bleed, direct pressure should be applied. Any continued bleeding can result in reduced oxygen carrying capacity.

4. (**A**) This patient needs the oxygen carrying capacity of red blood cells.

5. (**C**) Up and Over- the patient flies over the

wheel/dashboard fracturing both femurs (driver); then the thorax/abd impacts the wheel/dash causing trauma; then the face impacts the wheel/dash/windshield.

6. (**B**) The normal for hemoglobin is ~ 13-18 g/dL. The critical high/ low is > 20/< 7. Most texts will suggest replacing packed red blood cells after either 30% of blood loss has occurred or 7 g/dL or less HGB presents.

7. (**B**) High power weapons can bring with the projectile a pressure wave that can make the cranial vault explode. This is more likely to occur at closer ranges with high power firearms. However, this can occur with high power firearms at larger distances away, but in this case the high velocity/ close range answer is better because the fact that you're closer would cause more of an explosive effect.

8. (**D**) Up and Over- the patient flies over the wheel/dashboard fracturing both femurs (driver); then the thorax/abd impacts the wheel/dash causing trauma; then the face impacts the wheel/dash/windshield.

9. (**A**) Ultimately, this patient needs ventilation. The airway is open, so you do not need to reposition. Intubation is a method to ventilate, but just because you ventilate in an advanced form doesn't make it more correct. Suction, possible, but the question provides no information that there is fluid in the airway, so therefore, the most correct answer is Ventilation.

10. (**A**) Down and Under- the patient slides under the steering wheel or towards dashboard impacting knees causing knee, hip, and femur fxs; the chest strikes the wheel/dash causing thoracic and abd trauma; finally the head hits the wheel/ dash causing face and head trauma.

11. (**A**) Level 1 via Step 1 criteria (GCS < 13): He will not have a conversation with you, so yelling the same word over is inappropriate (-3), and not following commands/ combative (-1 for localizing your hands) brings the GCS to 11.

12. (**A**) The normal for hemoglobin is ~ 13-18 g/dL. The critical high/ low is > 20/< 7. This patient has lost a lot of fluid and has hemoconcentrated the blood and thus made the HGB high. Increase fluid resuscitation.

13. (**C**) Pale, mottled skin indicates a shock state. In the event of a stabbing, significant hemorrhage could occur and thus causing the skin to be shunted of blood.

14. (**C**) This is a traumatic asphyxia patient, and it is important to maintain hemodynamics. While it may be prudent to administer a buffering solution, like sodium bicarb, first have IV fluids ready and support the hemodynamics.

15. (**A**) Remember the s/s of splenic injury: Pain in LUQ and Kehr's Sign (left shoulder pain).

16. (**A**) This is a form of paralysis and thus meets Step II criteria for a LEVEL 1 trauma center.

17. (**C**) The mons pubis (pubic mound) is the tissue just above the vaginal opening. A laceration here with significant mechanism represents a pelvic fracture. Bind the pelvis is the best answer to prevent exsanguination.

18. (**C**) Bubbling indicates fluid in the airway- the first thing needed is suction.

19. (**D**) Remember the s/s of intestinal injury: abd pain, seatbelt sign, guarding, abdominal distension, rebound tenderness, vomiting, and fever.

20. (**D**) (1 unit = increase hemoglobin by 1 and increases hematocrit by 3). Therefore it should improve from 36% to 45%.

21. (**B**) If the patient has a high PTT, then it takes too long for their blood to clot- potentially due to over-aggressive anticoagulant therapy. Vitamin K is the reversal for warfarin, which is a blood thinner.

22. (**B**) With any antibiotics, allergy must be monitored, including uticaria, wheezing, and hypotension. Uticaria and wheezing represents localized effects, where hypotension represents systemic effects.

23. (**B**) The normal for hematocrit is ~ 40-55%, depending on gender. So, 11% is a critical low. A critical low would be a hematocrit 20% or less. A critical high is 65% or greater.

24. (**B**) (1 unit = increase hemoglobin by 1 and increases hematocrit by 3). Remember, 1 uint of PRBCs is typically 250 cc, so 500 cc makes up 2 units of PRBCs. Two units of PRBCs should increase the HGB from 10 g/dL to 12 g/dL.

25. (**E**) The normal for hematocrit is ~ 40-55%, depending on gender. So, 23% is low. A critical low would be a hematocrit 20% or less. A critical high is 65% or greater.

26. (**C**) The more blunt an object, the more difficult it is to cause penetration, therefore, more tissue crush is need to result in penetration. Each of these items are sharp except one: the baseball bat.

27. (**A**) An acetabular fracture is a type of hip/ pelvic fracture, so this meets Step 2 criteria and thus the patient should be taken to a Level I hospital.

28. (**B**) There is typically fluid in the smaller airways with pulmonary contusions because the tissue swells. Therefore, if we provide positive pressure ventilation or CPAP to push back that fluids trying to come out of lung tissue from the trauma. Pulmonary contusion best matches the treatment provided.

29. (**B**) The occlusive dressing isn't effective, and tension continues to build up in this patient. You need to needle decompress the chest and be ready to re-decompress throughout transport, or consider placing a chest tube. The other answer choices would not fix the problem.

30. (**A**) Kehr's sign classically indicates a splenic injury, but can also refer pain from an irritated diaphragm where the irritation is caused by blood. Kehr's Sign is typically manifests as left shoulder pain.

31. (**A**) Remember the s/s of rhabdo: dark colored urine, weakness/ dehydration, creatine kinase elevation (5 times normal), hyper K (>5.5mEq/L) with tall T waves on ECG, Hypocalcemia (<4.3mEq/L).

32. (**B**) Laying the bike down- massive road rash and unilateral extremity amputations/ fxs.

33. (**C**) (1 unit = increase hemoglobin by 1 and increases the hematocrit by 3). If given 3 units, the 7 g/dL should elevate to 10 g/dL.

34. (**B**) This patient has not been adequately resuscitated. For those of you stating you need more information, yes the

question would be easier if you had a baseline lactate, but if that patient had been there for over 4 hours and the lactate is still that high (normal 0.5-1 mmol/L), then you need to be suspicious of poor resuscitation. This patient needs aggressive fluid and blood product resuscitation.

35. (**C**) In this case the patient has a neurovascular compromise and the extremity needs to have traction and repositioning to try to establish perfusion.

36. (**A**) Down and Under- the patient slides under the steering wheel or towards dashboard impacting knees causing knee, hip, and femur fxs; the chest strikes the wheel/dash causing thoracic and abd trauma; finally the head hits the wheel/ dash causing face and head trauma.

37. (**B**) 1 unit of PRBSs raises HGB by 1 and raises HCT by 3. So, in this case, the HCT after blood administration should be 23%.

38. (**D**)The patient must have a high PTT, meaning it takes too long for his blood to clot and potentially due to aggressive of an anticoagulant therapy. Protamine sulfate is the reversal for heparin.

39. (**C**) There is no evidence here in favor for uterine or fetal injury, but Kehr's sign suggests a spleen injury (classically).

40. (**A**) Any pulseless extremity meets Step II criteria for a level 1 trauma center.

41. (**D**) Subcutaneous air along with clear and equal breath sounds point to a non- lung pathophysiology. Tracheobronchial injuries and laryngotracheal injuries all can allow air to collect subcutaneously. Additionally, the insult must be definitively corrected, so support ABCs and

get to a surgeon.

42. (**B**) Kehr's sign is present, but on the right side which indicates liver injury. Diaphragm irritation can also cause this, but if it were only a diaphragm injury, then most likely there wouldn't be shock present (pale skin). Kehr's Sign classically refers pain to the left shoulder, but also can point to the right shoulder in liver injuries. This is a little known fact. Focus on left should pain with Kehr's sign relating to splenic injury for these critical care certification exams.

43. (**A**) (1 unit = increase hemoglobin by 1 and increases hematocrit by 3). In this case, 2 units are given and therefore should raise the HCT from 19% to 25%.

44. (**B**) With asymmetrical chest wall in the absence of a flail segment (no paradoxical chest wall movement) then it is anticipated that there is a tension pneumothorax, thus needle decompression is immediately warranted. If you ventilate before decompressing, then you could worsen the tension.

45. (**D**) Dry and rattling is describing sonorous respirations, thus the tongue is falling to the back of the throat. Reposition the airway.

46. (**A**) In this case, there is evidence of a hip fracture (shortened leg) and therefore the hip needs to be bound to prevent significant hemorrhage into the pelvic cavity.

47. (**B**) This patient has mottled skin and poor capillary refill, which means they are experiencing shock (poor perfusion). The most important treatment is that which could improve perfusion: fluids is so important here. Of course, pressors can increase BP, but we stay away from them until we have to: fluids and blood first.

Trendelenburg has been found to not be beneficial and some literature suggests it is harmful.

48. (**A**) With any antibiotics, allergy must be monitored, including uticaria, wheezing, and hypotension. Uticaria and wheezing represents localized effects, where hypotension represents systemic effects.

49. (**B**) The normal for hemoglobin is ~ 13-18 g/dL. The critical high/ low is > 20/< 7. This patient has lost a lot of blood. Administer fluids including PRBCs or whole blood for their oxygen carrying capacity.

50. (**C**) Step 3 criteria include higher speed bicyclist vs. automobile (>20 mph) with being run-over.

51. (**D**) Here, the patient has fractures to ankles, hip and scaphoid fractures (wrists). Looks like this: Critical Fall: Calcaneus fx; tib/ fib, femur, and pelvic fxs; spinal fxs; bilateral colles' fxs; deceleration injuries (compression and shearing injuries).

52. (**D**) Lateral- these impacts result on unilateral extremity and pelvic fractures, head injuries from striking head against the impact side of the car, rotational injuries, etc.

53. (**C**) The information of broken 1st/ 2nd ribs (crepitus below the clavicle) and the difference in BP from the right or left arm, indicates an aortic rupture. Some of these other conditions can be present too, but this info REALLY points to aortic rupture.

54. (**D**) The giveaway here is the loss of pulse. This, in absence of crepitus, indicates increasing pressure within the compartment.

55. (**A**) Here, pulmonary contusions are present (young lungs with rales- rales due to damaged lung tissue). Therefore, it acts link acute lung injury/ ARDS, so higher PEEPs and pressure control modes are ideal. SIMV with PEEP at 10-15 is ideal per the current literature.

56. (**C**) This patient needs to improve perfusion, so ensure to support blood pressure aggressively and maximize oxygenation.

57. (**C**) High- risk auto crashes constitute a STEP 3 activation (ejection or partial ejection, death in the same vehicle).

58. (**A**) In this case, the patient doesn't meet criteria for Level I because the amputation was distal the ankle. Therefore, this patient needs to go to the closest appropriate facility.

59. (**A**) Permissive hypotension is a consideration when great vessel rupture is suggested, but here it is unclear if it is a great vessel injury, so go ahead and give fluids to target 90 systolic. Remember, these certification exams will try to trick you and sometimes you will need to choose the most correct answer even if it is a little off from what you studied. Like life, think in shades of grey instead of black vs. white.

60. (**D**) Cardiac Tamponade: Beck's triad, hypoxia syndrome, rising CVP (>15cm H2O), hypotension. These are all findings of cardiac tamponade.

61. (**A**) Myocardial contusion is characterized by ST elevation in leads II, III, and aVF with a wide QRS in V1 (BBB) especially in the face of direct chest trauma.

62. (**A**) A depressed skull fracture meets Step II criteria for a level 1 trauma center.

63. (**C**) If your trauma patient is on anticoagulants, then they most likely lost a ton of blood thus requiring them to receive anticoagulants in an attempt to minimize DIC.

64. (**B**) Checking plateau pressure isn't a bad idea, but only after ruling out tension pneumothorax, which is present here based on the alarm and chest asymmetry. Therefore, the best plan would be to needle decompress. Ventilating a tension pneumo could lead to death- decompress immediately.

65. (**C**) There must be bleeding still occurring, since the PRBCs did not correct the blood as expected (1 unit = increase hemoglobin by 1 and increases hematocrit by 3).

66. (**B**) Remember, the management for rahbdo is IV fluids- at least 2 L, 1mEq/kg bicarb, calcium q 5 minutes with ECG signs of hyperK, consider mannitol and adding bicarb to NS to alkalinize the urine (keep urine pH over 6.5).

67. (**C**) A hemothorax presents like this: hypoxia, hypotension, decreased BS to affected side, 'dull' chest percussion = hyporesonant, worsening shock, low CVP.

68. (**D**) Here a penetrating wound in the diaphragm is screaming at us that the person cannot breath because he cannot produce significant negative pressures under his diaphragm, thus cannot bring air into the lungs. Intubation is a method to ventilate, but just because you ventilate in an advanced form doesn't make it more correct. Good measure to always stick to less invasive management options, UNLESS the question asks for advanced management.

69. (**D**) That sharp back pain indicates an abruption. The shoulder pains also indicate bleeding, but the back pain is specific to an abruption.

70. (**D**) This patient needs to improve perfusion, so ensure to support blood pressure aggressively and maximize oxygenation.

71. (**A**) Absent heart tones (with a pulse) and JVD (with clear lung sounds) indicate cardiac tamponade, so a pericardiocentesis is needed. This procedure, simply stated, is removing fluid from the pericardial space.

72. (**B**) Secondary- Debris thrown from the blast; Primary- damage from the blast itself; Tertiary- patient becomes a missile; Quaternary- burning from building or collapsing wall of a building.

2 AIRCRAFT FUNDAMENTALS

Questions

1. Upon safely egressing the aircraft after a crash, you decide to return to the aircraft for survivors. You see a few small fires, but your partner insists "everything" was turned off and there isn't a chance of explosion. What is the most appropriate course of action next?

   A. Reinforce that the scene is not yet safe.
   B. Run to aircraft, retrieve survivors and egress.
   C. The scene is safe. Retrieve your crew from crash.
   D. The fire poses little danger. Retrieve your crew.

2. Following a crash, which of the following represents the correct shutdown procedure just prior egress?

   A. Throttle, Fuel, Batteries
   B. Throttle, Survival Kit, Batteries
   C. Survival Kit, Throttle, Fuel
   D. Batteries, Throttle, Fuel

3. After crashing, you are approaching the aircraft to look for and assist survivors. Which of the following, if observed, would cause you to retreat from the rescue attempt?

   A. Damage to the aircraft flight recorder
   B. Fire without evidence of spilled fuel
   C. Any secondary threat like bad weather
   D. A damaged main rotor that is not spinning

4. You are conducting a walk around prior to a flight. Which of these items pose a bigger danger?

   A. Air conditioner stored inside the hangar
   B. Electrical wires rolled up neatly near socket
   C. Rotor ties secured in the aft compartment
   D. Cowlings with fasteners in locked position

5. Which of the following is the correct procedure should the pilot have to make an emergency landing?

   A. Confirm emergency, relay info to dispatch, prep patient/ extra riders
   B. Unplug electrical devices, prep patient/ extra riders, inform dispatch
   C. Notify dispatch, inform pilot, relay info to dispatch, crash position
   D. Shut off throttle, fuel, and oxygen; inform dispatch; prep patient

6. You are approaching your landing zone. Which of the following is reasonable to request from the ground crew?

   A. Clear loose trash and articles from the LZ
   B. Instruct them to stand back 500 ft from LZ
   C. Have them hold the IV bag and line high
   D. Apply the back board to each patient

7. You need to exit the aircraft. What is the first thing you need to shut down upon egressing the aircraft?

   A. Oxygen
   B. The fuel
   C. Throttle
   D. Batteries

8. You find out that a helicopter crash that occurred a few months ago did not have their ELT triggered. This would alert the astute air transport clinician that

   A. the wreck occurred with an impact force of 3g
   B. the ELT must have been damaged during impact
   C. power to the ELT was disrupted during impact
   D. the force of impact in crash was greater than 5g

9. You are involved in a crash in a remote section of the country. Which of the main survival needs can be delayed in acquiring unless the rescuer will be estimated to take longer than 24 hours?

A. Signals
B. Shelter
C. Water
D. Fire

10. Upon exiting the aircraft following a crash, which of the following would be the most appropriate location to rendezvous with the remaining crew?

A. 200 ft from the front of the aircraft
B. 100 ft from the right of the aircraft
C. 125 ft from the aircraft tail rotor
D. 150 ft from the left of the aircraft

11. Which of the following would be important to request of the ground crew from a safety standpoint during your final approach to the landing zone?

A. Have them stand back 750 ft from LZ
B. Have them help place an airway
C. Pick up trash from the landing zone
D. Backboard all patients for transport

12. On the way to a call, you note the smell of smoke and identify a fire source. Which of the following is the first appropriate action?

A. Unplug the electrical devices
B. Use extinguisher to put out fire
C. Move away from the fire source
D. Notify the pilot immediately

13. You are on a scene flight and are returning to the aircraft with fire department assistants. The aircraft is running. Which of the following actions should you take as you approach a running helicopter?

A. Maintain the IV drips high to optimize gravity flow
B. Send the first responders to the aircraft without you
C. Continue sterile cockpit standards as you approach
D. Keep eye contact with the pilot for their directions

14. Which of the following situations would it be reasonable to abort a flight?

A. Crew member needing to get off on time to meet family
B. Pilot who has 5 hours of duty time and a 1 hour flight
C. Nighttime NVG flight with 2000ft/ 5 miles over mountains
D. Your partner who just doesn't feel good about flight

15. If a fire breaks out while in flight, what is the correct in-flight procedure for this issue?

A. Notify pilot, unplug electrical devices, utilize fire extinguisher
B. Notify pilot, utilize fire extinguisher, unplug electrical devices
C. Unplug electrical devices, utilize fire extinguisher, notify pilot
D. Unplug electrical devices, notify pilot, utilize fire extinguisher

16. It is dusk and you on in flight and on your way to a patient. You are now focusing on your LZ. Which of the following represents adequate landing zones?

A. 120x120 anytime; 100x100 night time
B. 60x60 night time and 100x100 anytime
C. 50x50 day time; 60x60 night time
D. 60x60 day time and 75x75 night time

17. You are standing outside your aircraft as the spotter while the aircraft is shutting down. From which direction is the most dangerous to approach a rotor wing aircraft?

A. 11 o'clock
B. 2 o'clock
C. 7 o'clock
D. 12 o'clock

18. While on a night mission, you are performing high recon of the LZ. Which of the following represents an adequate landing zone?

A. 100x100 ft on a flat surface
B. 60x60 without garbage in LZ
C. 50x50 but with a spotter
D. 75x75 with an "X" in lights

19. This is the best instructions to give to ground crew members assisting you to transition a patient to a rotor-turning aircraft?

A. Slide chart in between the patient's legs
B. Lower head and hold the IV poles high
C. Tighten up hat straps when near aircraft
D. Be sure to tightly hold onto loose items

20. Which of the following meets minimum weather standards as per CAMTS?

A. 750 ft and 1 mile, day time, cross country, over mountains with NVGs
B. 900 ft and 3.2 miles locally non-mountainous at night with NVGs
C. 1250 ft and 2 miles, night, locally, over mountains, without NVG
D. 1000 ft and 3 miles cross country over mountains at night without NVGs

21. Ground crew helpers are helping you get the patient back to your helicopter for a hot on-load. What would be some good things to communicate to the ground crew prior to approaching the aircraft?

A. Hold on tightly to items people are carrying
B. Push paperwork under the head of stretcher
C. Always keep IV poles high above the patient
D. Wear hats snuggly and look pilot in eyes

22. An FAA report of a helicopter crash states that the ELT was not activated. Which of the following must be true?

A. The ELT had malfunctioned
B. The ELT had a loss of power
C. The impact was less than 4g
D. the force damaged the ELT

23. During flight, the pilot states he has to make an emergency landing. What is the most appropriate first step in emergency procedures during this situation?

A. Confirm the emergency
B. prep patient & extra riders
C. Unplug electrical devices
D. Relay info to dispatch

24. Upon approaching the aircraft on a scene to load the patient into the aircraft with the help of assistants, which of the following ground assistants should cause you to stop and correct the error?

A. The assistant with his hat backwards to prevent it from flying off
B. The sheriff's deputy who in his squad car and with the door closed
C. The EMT who is ducking while he is helping to push the stretcher
D. Your partner who has his helmet on their head making eye contact

25. Describe the term "sterile cockpit".

A. Term used to describe the silence invoked during takeoff and landing and other critical phases of flight
B. Term used to describe the silence invoked during critical medical procedures and critical phases of care
C. Term used to describe the silence invoked during radio traffic and critical phases of communication
D. Term used to describe the silence invoked from takeoff to landing allowing the pilot to concentrate at all times

26. You are in cruise flight and notice an obstacle that the aircraft could hit within a few seconds. Which of the following reflects the best way to communicate this to the pilot?

A. "11 o'clock low. Radio tower. Abort."
B. "Radio antenna. Abort right. 11 o'clock low."
C. "Abort! 11 o'clock low. Radio tower."
D. "Abort right. Radio tower. 11 o'clock low."

27. You are in the aircraft performing high recon of the LZ. Which of the following would pose the largest threat upon landing?

A. Knee high grass in the LZ
B. Power line 30ft from the LZ
C. Fire trucks 150 away from LZ
D. Strobe lights at the LZ

28. You are in cruise flight and notice an obstacle that the aircraft could hit within a few seconds. Which of the following reflects the best way to communicate this to the pilot?

A. "Abort! Abort! 10 o'clock low. water tank."
B. "High antenna! Abort! It is at 10 o'clock."
C. "Abort right! Antenna wire. 2 o'clock low."
D. "12 o'clock low. Water tower. Abort."

29. As you approach a scene, the pilot asks you to look for hazards in the LZ. An astute flight clinician recognizes the following as potential hazards to the aircraft:

A. A police office 100 ft away in his vehicle
B. Approaching aircraft form downhill side
C. Ground strobe lights and short fences
D. A baseball cap on a first responder's head

30. From which direction is it most unsafe to approach the aircraft?

A. From the front
B. The pilots left side
C. Pilot's right side
D. From the backside

31. You crash in a remote forest in February in the northwest part of the country. What is the first thing you need to do?

A. Obtain food
B. Build a shelter
C. Obtain water
D. Build a camp fire

32. You crash on a grassy plain in the Midwest. As you egress, what should be your first action in reference to shutting down the engine?

   A. Cut off the fuel supply
   B. Shut off the oxygen
   C. Pull the throttle back
   D. Turn off the batteries

Answers

1. (**A**) It is acceptable to return to the aircraft for survivors once all primary threats are gone. Primary threats would include lingering moving parts, fire and explosion. Therefore, the correct answer is DO NOT APPROACH. The fire could spark explosion.

2. (**A**) The correct procedure is throttle, fuel, and batteries to best reduce the chance of fire.

3. (**B**) It is acceptable to return to the aircraft for survivors once all primary threats are gone. Primary threats would include lingering moving parts, **fire** and explosion. Therefore, the correct answer is B because it includes fire. The fire could spark explosion.

4. (**C**) Prior to your shift and prior to each flight, you should do a walk around to include looking for loose debris, as well as cords, cowlings, covers to all be in their appropriate positions and locations. ALL cowlings should be in there locked down position. It is OK to have rolled up like school wires near a socket place they are based on FAA regulations. Rotor tie securely fastened to the aircraft is appropriate from time to time, but obviously you would need to remove these before flight.

5. (**A**) The correct procedure is help the pilot confirm the emergency, relay any information to dispatch that is important, shut off the power and oxygen, and prepare the patient and crew for a crash.

6. (**A**) The best answer here is to clear the debris from a safety standpoint and with respect to communications with the ground crew. The IV and backboard answer selections are incorrect because they deal with patient treatment and not safety. Having them stand back 500ft is an excessive distance and is impractical in several scenarios.

7. (**C**) The appropriate procedure is to shut off the throttle, fuel, and then batteries. This reduces the chance of fire.

8. (**A**) ELTs are very tough devices, and thus their being damaged isn't likely. If the ELT wasn't damaged, then the impact must have been under 4g, therefore, the "the wreck occurred with an impact force of 3g" is the correct answer.

9. (**C**) We can go 3 days without water, so it can be delayed unless the estimated rescue time is greater than 24 hours. This is so you'd have 2 day to look for water. Important to not wait until the 3 day to begin looking for water. But we can die in cold weather within 3 hours without shelter and fire.

10. (**A**) The first location to meet up after a crash is at the 12 o'clock position. As an alternative, you could meet up at the 3 and 9 o'clock positions. The 6 o'clock position is relatively unsafe as the tail rotor could still rotating and causing a danger.

11. (**C**) The best answer here is to pick up trash from a safety standpoint and with respect to communications with the ground crew. The airway and backboard answer selections are incorrect because they deal with patient treatment and not safety. Having them stand back 750ft is an excessive distance and is impractical in several scenarios.

12. (**D**) The correct procedure per textbook is notify pilot, utilize fire extinguisher, unplug electrical devices.

13. (**D**) You always need to keep eye contact with the pilot while walking to the aircraft with others. Keep eye contact with the assistants too to prevent them from doing something that could cause harm to the crew or assistants.

14. (**D**) For any reason, real or perceived, a crew member can turn down a flight. A crew member needing to get off on time has nothing to do with safety. A 1 hour flight and 5 hours of duty time (or the remaining time the FAA says they can fly) also doesn't have anything to do with safety. The CAMTS weather minimums are safe and acceptable for a flight. The only one that is safety related is the "perceived" danger the crewmember of feels. It is legitimate to decline a flight based on actual or perceived mechanical or other issues.

15. (**B**) The correct procedure per textbook is notify pilot, utilize fire extinguisher, unplug electrical devices.

16. (**A**) Appropriate LZ features include a 60 by 60 foot flat surface with minimal high obstructions and minimal debris for day time operations and for night time operations a 100 by 100 foot flat surface with minimal high obstructions and minimal debris is desired. Therefore, the correct answer is 120x120 anytime and 100x100 night time satisfies both day and night dimension requirements.

17. (**C**) Rotor wing aircrafts should never be approached from the 6 o'clock position, or any directions similar to the 6 o'clock position (which includes 4-8 o'clock). With the main rotors running, people do not notice the tail rotor and will walk right into it. Additionally, we cannot make

eye contact with the pilot who may need to alert us to something important. Therefore, the correct answer is 8 o'clock because it is too close to the 6 o'clock direction.

18. (**A**) Appropriate LZ features include a 60 by 60 foot flat surface with minimal high obstructions and minimal debris for day time operations and for night time operations a 100 by 100 foot flat surface with minimal high obstructions and minimal debris is desired. Therefore, the correct answer is 100x100 which satisfies the dimension requirements.

19. (**D**) Never trust anything loose that you do not have a hand on, therefore, tucking the chart and wearing hats snuggly answer selections are incorrect. Never hold anything high, therefore, the IV pole answer selection is also incorrect. The best answer here is to grasp x-rays tightly and have the ground crew to remove their hats.

20. (**B**) The only one that is under weather minimums is 900 ft and 3.2 miles locally non-mountainous at night with NVGs. It is important to know these weather minimums- you will get 1-2 questions on your exam concerning these minimums.

21. (**A**) Never trust anything loose that you do not have a tight grip on, therefore, tucking the chart and wearing hats snuggly answer selections are incorrect. Never hold anything high, therefore, the IV pole answer selection is also incorrect. The best answer here is to grasp x-rays tightly and have the ground crew to remove their hats.

22. (**C**) The ELT requires 4g to become activated.

23. (**A**) The correct procedure is help the pilot confirm the emergency, relay any information to dispatch that is

important, shut off the power and oxygen, and prepare the patient and crew for a crash.

24. (**A**) To keep the scene safe , you will have to keep other safe who do not have the training you have. That includes keeping the untrained from making mistakes including loose clothing, hats, lose sheets, and holding IV poles high around the aircraft while it is running. Here the biggest concern is backwards hat which could still fly off the first responder's head.

25. (**A**) This is the concept that everyone is quiet and looking outside the aircraft during critical phases of flight (taxi, takeoff, and landing).

26. (**D**) In this case, telling a pilot where to go FIRST ("Abort right") could save your life. Therefore, this is the most correct answer.

27. (**B**) A true hazard is one that poses a DIRECT threat to the aircraft. While it is true that indirect threats (ones that could lead to a threat to the aircraft, like shining a light in the pilot's eyes) could be argued to be 'potential hazards', the most correct answers are those that pose direct threats. Therefore, the correct answer is power lines because it could damage the aircraft- the power line can be struck causing the aircraft to crash. The others are not a direct threat.

28. (**C**) In this case, telling a pilot where to go FIRST ("Abort right" could save your life. The pilot will instinctively trust you and head in that direction. Therefore, this is the most correct answer.

29. (**D**) A true hazard is one that poses a DIRECT threat to the aircraft. While it is true that indirect threats (ones that

could lead to a threat to the aircraft, like shining a light in the pilot's eyes) could be argued to be 'potential hazards', the most correct answers are those that pose direct threats. Therefore, the correct answer is the hat that could come off of the first responders head and damage aircraft components.

30. (**D**) Rotor wing aircrafts should never be approached from the 6 o'clock position or rear when the rotors are turning, or any directions similar to the 6 o'clock position (which includes 2-8 o'clock). With the main rotors running, people do not notice the tail rotor and will walk right into it. Additionally, we cannot make eye contact with the pilot who may need to alert us to something important. Therefore, the correct answer is 8 o'clock because it is too close to the 6 o'clock direction.

31. (**B**) The correct order of post-crash priorities is shelter, fire, and then food. Water becomes an issue if the rescue takes longer than 24 hours.

32. (**C**) The appropriate procedure is to shut off the throttle, fuel, and then batteries. This best reduces the chance of fire.

3 FLIGHT PHYSIOLOGY

Questions

1. During a shift briefing, your pilot mentions there are several mountains in the area and going over them will diminish your night vision by half. You recognize the altitudes you'll be flying will be greater than _______.

   A. 1000
   B. 2000
   C. 3000
   D. 4000

2. Your patient is exhibiting chest pain; (+) ST elevation in II, III, and aVF; JVD, and SpO2 is 86%. What type of hypoxia is present?

   A. Hypoxic
   B. Hypemic
   C. Stagnant
   D. Histotoxic

3. Your ventilator patient has become hypoxic. You adjust the FiO2 to obtain better SpO2. You recall this is because of which of the following gas laws?

   A. Fick's Law
   B. Boyle's Law
   C. Charles' Law
   D. Henry's Law

4. You apply a pulse oximeter to a patient and obtain the following: HR 105 and oxygen saturations 90%. This identifies which of the following conditions?

   A. Hyperoxemia
   B. Hypoxia
   C. Hypoxemia
   D. Euoxcemia

5. You depart for a rotorwing mountain rescue at approximately 17,500 ft. Which of the following is true?

   A. You will have 20 minutes of EPT.
   B. You will have 40 minutes of TUC.
   C. You will have 10 minutes of EPT.
   D. You will have 5 minutes of TUC.

6. You intubated a patient on scene who was bagged prior to your arrival. You take off from sea level and have to fly over a 9500 foot peak. At this altitude, the patient experiences a high pressure alarm. What is the cause?

   A. Boyle's law- from abdominal distention
   B. Charles' law- higher temperatures
   C. Fick's law- Air is denser at altitude
   D. Henry's law- partial pressures change

7. You are at 30,000 ft and you recall that your TUC is about 1 minute. What would your EPT be should you experience a cabin decompression?

   A. 120 seconds
   B. 4 minutes
   C. 1 second
   D. 8 minutes

8. Your awake patient experiences a grand mal seizure while in flight. Which of the following stressors of flight can cause this to occur?

   A. Dehydration
   B. Flicker vertigo
   C. Third Spacing
   D. Vibration

9. Before flight on a January evening in Illinois, your skid-mounted oxygen tank measured 1800 PSI, but at altitude its 1650 PSI. You have not administered any oxygen yet. Which gas law explains this difference?

A. Charles
B. Fick's
C. Gay-Lussacs
D. Hennery's

10. When transporting a patient from Tampa, FL to Denver, CO, you calculate you'll have to increase the FiO2 setting from 0.5 to 0.7. You recognize that this was based on which of the following gas laws?

A. Graham's Law
B. Dalton's Law
C. Gay-Lussac's
D. Charles' Law

11. Your patient's ABG returns and reflects a pO2 of 51 mmHg. This indicates which of the following conditions?

A. Hypoxia
B. Hyperoxia
C. Euoxia
D. Hypoxemia

12. A patient was assaulted with a sledgehammer with impacts to the chest and abdomen. He is short of breath and presents with JVD and distant heart tones. What is the cause of their hypoxia?

    A. Hypoxic
    B. Hypemic
    C. Histotoxic
    D. Stagnant

13. You just learned that O2 diffuses slower than molecular carbon dioxide across a membrane. This is explained by which gas law?

    A. Dalton's Law
    B. Henry's Law
    C. Graham's Law
    D. Charles' Law

14. When air transporting a patient with shortness of breath following a deep SCUBA dive, a sudden onset of a dry uncontrollable cough and a feeling of suffocation indicates which gas law as the prime culprit?

    A. Charles' Law
    B. Boyle's Law
    C. Henry's Law
    D. Gay-Lussac's

15. Which of the following are stressors of flight that are effected by altitude?

    A. Barometric pressure/ dehydration/ third spacing
    B. Effects of vibration/ third spacing/ hypoxia/ Noise
    C. Special disorientation/ thermal/ hypoxia/ fatigue
    D. Noise/ special disorientation/ vibration/thermal

16. After a long shift where you were in the air for a total of 6 hours over 4 flights you feel extremely exhausted despite resting and taking in appropriate nutrition. What is causing your exhaustion?

    A. From dehydration
    B. Fatigue from vibration
    C. Hypoxia from altitude
    D. From hypoglycemia

17. A patient is experiencing difficulty breathing after an inhalation burn and their pulse oximetry reads 100%. Why is this patient short of breath?

    A. They are histotoxically hypoxic
    B. They are hypemically hypoxic
    C. They are stagnantly hypoxic
    D. They are hypoxically hypoxic

18. You leave Seattle (760 torr) heading for Denver (620). Your intubated patient is on 0.8 FiO2. How will you manage this patient's oxygenation needs?

    A. Increase the FiO2 to 80%
    B. Increase the FiO2 to 90%
    C. Increase the FiO2 to 98%
    D. No changes are needed.

19. As you ascend from city A to city B, the barometric pressure reduces from 721 mmHg in City A to 625 in City B. You will use this information to calculate a corrected FiO2 for your intubated patient. What gas law does this pertain to?

    A. Boyles
    B. Grahams
    C. Daltons
    D. Charles

20. While in a critical phase of flight, your partner complains of an earache. Which of the critical phases of flight would this occur?

    A. Taxiing
    B. Landing
    C. Take-off
    D. Sharp turn

21. In flight, you hear a high pressure alarm from the ventilator. You're patient's blood pressure and pulse oximetry dramatically fall acutely. You make note that you are at 8500 ft. Which gas law explains this change?

    A. Boyles
    B. Daltons
    C. Gay-Lussacs
    D. Charles

22. Your patient drops their SpO2. You attempt to improve oxygenation by increasing the PEEP setting. You recall this is because of which of the following gas laws?

    A. Henry's Law
    B. Boyle's Law
    C. Charles' Law
    D. Fick's Law

23. Upon a rapid decompression in a fixed-wing aircraft, the pilot mentions you are at FL 240. How long do you have before you go unconsciousness if you do not apply oxygen?

    A. about 2 minutes
    B. about 30 seconds
    C. about 5 seconds
    D. About 5 minutes

24. You have a patient that is choking on a piece of food, is becoming cyanotic, and their pulse oximetry reads 87%. What type of hypoxia is present?

    A. Hypoxic
    B. Hypemic
    C. Stagnant
    D. Histotoxic

25. While en route to pick up a patient, your partner begins falling asleep despite attempts to remain awake. Fifteen minutes earlier, they were behaving fine. At what altitude range would you assess you currently were based on this information?

    A. Below 5K
    B. 10-14K
    C. 8-12K
    D. Above 15K

26. You land at an altitude of 12,500 ft and will be delayed taking off. Which of the following stages of hypoxia would you be experiencing?

    A. Compensatory stage
    B. Indifferent stage
    C. Disturbance stage
    D. Critical stage

27. During a night flight, your pilot becomes suddenly concerned and banks the aircraft hard. He states he needs to 'right' the aircraft although the horizontal compass is at a 45 degree slant. This could indicate which of the following?

A. Special disorientation
B. An episode of fatigue
C. Severe flicker vertigo
D. Hypoxia & dehydration

28. You transition your patient from the aircraft to the ER at a higher altitude than where you retrieved the patient. From which stressor are you suffering?

A. Third spacing
B. Flicker vertigo
C. Barometric pressure
D. Hypemic hypoxia

29. An infant develops a tension pneumothorax while at 7500 ft. Which gas law explains this?

A. Dalton's Law
B. Charles' Law
C. Fick's Law
D. Boyle's Law

30. A patient you are caring for has the following vital signs: HR 99, BP 118/72, pO2 is 50 mHg. Which of the following most accurately describes the current condition?

    A. Low HGB
    B. Hypoxia
    C. Hypoxemia
    D. Low RBCs

31. Upon assessing a patient you note an oxygen saturation of 84%. What does this value suggest?

    A. Reduced oxygen carrying capacity
    B. The patient has reduced hemoglobin
    C. Massive hemorrhage has occurred
    D. Decreased oxygen at distal tissues

32. Upon waking up in the morning while at an altitude much higher than where you live, you have very dry mucous membranes. You recall this is caused by which stressor?

    A. Fatigue
    B. Vibration
    C. Third Spacing
    D. Low humidity

33. Your patient is on high dose nitrates status post cath lab. Reportedly, the patient had very little heart damage, they are profoundly hypoxic. What type of hypoxia is present?

A. Stagnant
B. Hypoxic
C. Hypemic
D. Histotoxic

34. You are transporting a trauma patient in the winter where you forget to put a blanket on the patient. Which of the following conditions is currently effecting this patient?

A. Severe low oxygen in blood
B. Increased oxygen to tissues
C. Left oxyhemoglobin shift
D. Right oxyhemoglobin shift

Answers

1. (**D**) Night vision will decrease by 50% at approximately 4000ft in MSL.

2. (**C**) The problem here is a pump problem from the AMI. An AMI damages the heart and thus it cannot pump well, so fluid backs up into the jugular vein (JVD). No pulmonary edema is present so therefore it isn't a hypoxic hypoxia problem because oxygen has good access to the alveolar capillary membrane. The evidence of a poor pump indicates blood is not being pumped forward efficiently- therefore this is a STAGNANT hypoxia problem.

3. (A) Fick's Law says that if you increase the partial pressure of oxygen (via increasing FiO2), then oxygenation will improve (measured by O2 saturations). It also says that by increasing the surface area of a membrane and making the membrane thinner (both achieved via PEEP) then oxygenation also improves. Basically, Fick's says that by applying increased FiO2 and PEEP, you will obtain higher oxygen saturations.

4. (**B**) Hypoxia describes a lack of oxygen at the tissues. A pulse oximeter shines a red light onto red blood cells and estimates how saturated with oxygen they are. The pulse oximeter typically is placed on the skin which is a distal tissue. Therefore, hypoxia is a lack of oxygen at the TISSUES.

5. (**A**) At about 18,000 ft (close to 17,500 ft), you will have about 20-30 minutes of EPT and 10-15 of TUC. Therefore, the best answer is 20 minutes of EPT. Also, in rotor wing, we will always be dealing with EPT since we do not pressurize our cabins. There is no chance for "sudden" decompression.

6. (**A**) Boyle's Law states that gases will expand at altitude, therefore, suctioning the gut with a NGT or OGT is common practice to prevent a buildup of air in the stomach which could compress on the diaphragm and cause higher PIPs leading to a high pressure alarm.

7. (**A**) Remember that EPT is double that of TUC. Said another way, TUC is half of the bigger value, EPT. If you half EPT, you'll arrive at a good estimate of the TUC. In this case, double the TUC (1 minute) to arrive at the EPT (2 minutes, which is the same as 120 seconds).

8. (**B**) In a rotor wing aircraft, flicker vertigo is possible because light coming through the rotating blades is between 4-20/ sec. This has been shown to cause seizures in some individuals. It is important to pay close attention to seizure risk patient's during the day on helicopters.

9. (**C**) Gay-Lussacs law explains that as you go higher in altitude you will get colder because lower pressure translates into colder temperatures. This is commonly confused for Charles's Law which says that if you heat air up at a particular altitude, it expands, like in a hot air balloon. So, needing a jacket at altitude then is due to Gay-Lussac's Law.

10. (**B**) Recall that Dalton's Law states the total pressure of a gas is equal to the sum of its individual pressures. Therefore, you can use this to calculate the required oxygen needs if you knew your beginning and ending altitudes. FiO2 at destination = [(P1)(FiO2@takeoff)/(P2)], where P1 = the barometric pressure at takeoff and P2 is the barometric pressure at landing.

11. (**D**) Hypoxemia describes a lack of oxygen within the blood. It is a direct measure of the oxygen tension (partial pressure of oxygen) within the blood. If it is lower than 80 mmHg, then hypoxemia is present.

12. (**D**) This patient is experiencing a textbook cardiac tamponade. They would, therefore, have hypoxia based on the poor blood flow caused by the tamponade. This is termed STAGNANT hypoxia.

13. (**C**) Graham's law says that lighter molecules diffuse faster than heavier molecules, therefore, Graham's Law is the correct answer.

14. (**C**) This law describes lower atmospheric pressure = gas wanting to come out of a solution and collect in anatomical areas. Therefore, the correct answer in this case is Henry's Law- the backbone of decompression illness.

15. (**A**) The 6 stressors of flight that are relative to altitude are hypoxia, pressure, fatigue, thermal, dehydration, and third spacing. The 5 non-flight dependent stressor are noise, vibration, gravitational forces, special disorientation, and flicker vertigo.

16. (**B**) Vibration causes movement (shaking) and the body will attempt to keep you in one spot. Over several hours of flying, you will be very tired from the prolonged effort of your body to keep you in one spot.

17. (**A**) The inhalation burn with 100% sats and breathing difficulty suggests carbon monoxide poisoning. Therefore, this is a histotoxic problem.

18. (**C**) Recall this can be calculated by the equation: [(pressure at liftoff) x(FiO2)] / (pressure at altitude)]. Therefore, [(760) x(0.8)] / (620)] = 0.98.

19. (**C**) Dalton's law is the law of the sum of partial pressures. So, we can use the barometric pressure of a city and multiply it by our administered FiO2 and figure out the partial pressure of oxygen we are delivering to the patient. Additionally, we can set up a simple equation (see page 42) to calculate how much to increase FiO2 at our destination to ensure we are delivering the correct partial pressure of oxygen to our patients.

20. (**C**) Barodentalgia occurs during ascent when Boyles law says that gases expand as you go higher. Air thus expands in tooth cavities causing a great deal of pain- and this occurs during ASCENT, or take-off.

21. (**A**) As you go up in altitude, the weight of the atmosphere is decreasing and thus gasses are allowed to spread out. At sea level, the entire atmosphere is forcing gas molecules to stay close to one another. IT appears a pneumothorax has manifested.

22. (D) Fick's Law says that if you increase the partial pressure of oxygen (via increasing FiO2), then oxygenation will improve (measured by O2 saturations). It also says that by increasing the surface area of a membrane and making the membrane thinner (both achieved via PEEP) then oxygenation also improves. Basically, Fick's says that by applying increased FiO2 and PEEP, you will obtain higher oxygen saturations.

23. (**A**) This is a sudden decompression, so the better measurement is the TUC. In this case, at 25,000 ft, you'll have 1.5 - 3.5 minutes without oxygen.

24. (**A**) An obstruction here is blocking a sufficient amount of oxygen from gaining access to the alveolar capillary membrane. Therefore, this is a hypoxic problem.

25. (**D**) This patient situation is consistent with the disturbance stage of hypoxia. The patient is behaving as if he is drunk within a short time after entering a hypoxic environment. The disturbance stage is between 15-20K feet.

26. (**A**) This elevation is consistent with the compensatory stage of hypoxia. The disturbance stage is between 15-20K feet, the indifferent stage is between 5-12K feet, and the critical stage is above 20K feet.

27. (**A**) In flight, we receive conflicting information so disorientation can occur easily. This occurs when the pilot is under an illusion of intense movement of the aircraft (when actually the aircraft is in level flight) and in turn makes a drastic in course to correct the perceived problem. This can quickly result in a crash as the aircraft goes from level flight into a dive or into terrain (aka Type

III special disorientation).

28. (**C**) At higher altitudes (lower barometric pressure), there is less oxygen, thus energy cannot be produced in normal quantities, therefore fatigue occurs much faster at altitude than at sea level. Therefore, barometric pressure is the correct answer.

29. (**D**) Boyle's Law describes the inverse relationship between Volume and Pressure. Thus, higher altitudes = lower atmospheric pressure = gas expands.

30. (**C**) The pO2 is a direct measurement of the oxygen bound to hemoglobin and is a very specific test. It is NOT hypoxia, because hypoxia estimates reduced oxygen content in the cells, not in the blood. This is the biggest difference between hypoxia and hypoxemia- hypoxemia is low oxygen in the BLOOD while hypoxia is low oxygen in the TISSUES. This is a common misnomer and a favorite of test writers to try and trip you up.

31. (**D**) Reduced HGB, blood loss, and carrying capacity all are describing the same thing and are wrong in this case. Pulse oximetry simply explains the saturation of RBCs and estimates the amount of oxygen getting to the distal tissues.

32. (**D**) At altitude, there is much less moisture in the air. Therefore, at altitude, you are prone to dehydration. You should drink extra water to prevent dehydration due to low humidity.

33. (**D**) This is a tough question. To answer this question you have to know that high dose NITRATES can cause cyanide

toxicity. If you knew that, then the answer is clear (histotoxic hypoxia) and this supported since their heart wasn't damaged (r/o stagnant hypoxia).

34. (**C**) Hypothermia causes a left shift in the oxyhemoglobin dissociation curve. This means that oxygen VERY strongly sticks to the RBCs- so much (in hypothermia) that when the oxygenated RBC gets to the tissues, it doesn't let it go. If a RBC doesn't release oxygen to the tissues, then acidosis occurs.

4 AIRWAY

Questions

1. Before intubation via RSI you observe the following, HR 110, BP 88/61, RR 22, SpO2 96%, pH 7.38, pCO2 41. Which of the following medication sequences would be appropriate?

   A. Versed, Etomidate, Ketamine
   B. Rocuronium, ketamine, succinylcholine
   C. Succinylcholine, ketamine, versed
   D. Ketamine, succinylcholine, zemuron

2. Your adult trauma patient is intubated and has the following ventilator settings: A/C, RR 11, VT 460, FIO2 100%, PEEP 4. His vital signs are BP 124/76, HR 70, SPO2 98%, ETCO2 52. The next most appropriate action is to?

   A. Raise the RR to 14
   B. Adjust the Vt to 425
   C. Adjust the PEEP to 6
   D. Reduce FiO2 to 0.7

3. An adult trauma patient requires intubation. Which of the following would maximize pre-oxygenation efforts during the preparation phase of intubation?

   A. Lay the patient flat with BVM ventilations
   B. Squeeze the bag gently during BVM breaths
   C. Bag the patient with a PEEP valve attached
   D. Ensure the patient's chin is to their chest

4. Which of the following patients represents an indication for a surgical airway?

   A. You can't place the ETT and BVM ventilations results in SpO2 of 83%
   B. The patient has copious amounts of vomitus in their posterior oropharynx
   C. The patient has suffered a traumatic brain injury with motor deficits
   D. The patient is a COPD patient and has a tracheal surgical scar

5. Your pediatric patient weighing approximately 27 kg presents with an altered level of consciousness and you decide to intubate to protect their airway. Which of the following medications is appropriate for this patient?

   A. 27 mcg of Ketamine
   B. 0.54 mg Atropine
   C. 0.12 mg Rocuronium
   D. 27 mg of Fentanyl

6. Your adult difficulty breathing patient began developing respiratory failure and you decide to intubate. Vitals: HR 104, RR 24, BP 92/40. They are wheelchair bound, but can normally move all extremities. Which of the following RSI regimens is appropriate?

   A. Versed, Succinylcholine, Rocuronium
   B. Fentanyl, Ketamine, Rocuronium
   C. Vecuronium, Fentanyl, Succinylcholine
   D. Versed, Rocuronium, Fentanyl

7. Which of the following patients would best benefit from an RSI regimen of Ketamine, Rocuronium, and Fentanyl?

   A. 6 y/o asthmatic with increasing EtCO2
   B. AMI patient with altered mental status
   C. 72 y/o stroke patient with a very high ICP
   D. Trauma patient a tension pneumothorax

8. Currently, your adult patient is intubated with a 7.0 ETT, and secured with a commercial device at 25 at the gum line. Their vital signs are as follows: HR 121, BP is 108/74, SpO2 is 88%, and their EtCO2 is 54. Which of the following is the best immediate action?

   A. Reduce the MV
   B. Increase the FiO2
   C. Back up the ETT
   D. Increase the HOB

9. Your medical patient requires intubation. Your patient has the current labs and vitals: HR 105, BP 90/72, RR 22, SpO2 90%, pH 7.38, pCO2 38. Which of the following medication sequences would be appropriate?

   A. Ativan, Etomidate, Ketamine
   B. Zemuron, ketamine, succinylcholine
   C. Anectine, ketamine, versed
   D. Ketamine, Anectine, zemuron

10. Your medical patient presented lying face down on the ground and vomiting. Upon deep painful stimulation the patient withdraws their hand, but does not open their eyes. The patient also did not make any sounds when painful stimuli was applied. Which of the following procedures is most appropriate?

    A. nasal cannula placed
    B. Tracheal intubation
    C. OPA adjunct placed
    D. BVM ventilations

11. You are caring for a seriously injured patient. During your patient assessment, you find that the patient has a decreased level of consciousness, an absent gag reflex, and a poor response to painful stimuli. Based on this information, which of the following interventions would be most appropriate?

    A. A tracheostomy
    B. Endotracheal intubation
    C. Oral suctioning
    D. Nasal pharyngeal airway

12. While evaluating a 5 month old 7 kg patient with RSV, you decide it is best to protect his airway. You note retractions, pale and warm skin, and their capillary refill time is 4 seconds. Which of the following RSI regimens would be most appropriate?

A. Atropine 0.14, Ketamine 10 mg, Anectine 14 mg
B. Atropine 0.14, Versed 1 mg, Rocuronium 14 mg
C. Atropine 0.28, Ketamine 10 mcg, Anectine 0.28 mg
D. Atropine 0.28, Versed 0.1 mg, Rocuronium 28 mg

13. Your patient suffered 90% full and partial thickness burns 4 days ago. Their current vitals are BP 99/62, HR 101, SpO2 90%. What is the ideal RSI regime?

A. Versed, succinylcholine, rocuronium
B. Ketamine, succinylcholine, pancurionium
C. Etomidate, Fentanyl, zemuron,
D. Morphine, Anectine, rocuronium

14. You arrive just after a patient has been intubated in a small ER. As you are receiving the report, the x- ray return and shows the left lung fields to be completely white, HR is 118, BP is 115/55, EtCO2 is 51, and the SpO2 is 87%. Which of the following is the best immediate action?

A. Set a higher targeted VE
B. Apply the max of FiO2
C. Reposition the ET tube
D. Lower the patients head

15. Your medical patient is experiencing a PE. This would be considered to be which of the following?

    A. Oxygenation problem
    B. Ventilation problem
    C. Poor cardiac output
    D. Increased tachycardia

16. Succinylcholine is contraindicated in which of the following patients?

    A. New CVA patient with left sided weakness
    B. An AMI patent with antiplatelet on board
    C. The patient who's been bed bound 3 weeks
    D. Trauma patient with severe hypotension

17. Your patient has a nasal EtCO2 detector, and you notice a 'shark fin' pattern on the EtCO2 graphic waveform. You have made the decision to intubate the patient. Which of the following RSI regimens would be ideal?

    A. Succinylcholine, ketamine
    B. Lorazepam, zemuron
    C. Midazolam, etomidate
    D. Etomidate, rocuronium

18. Your 100 kg adult sepsis patient is awaiting transport to a larger regional facility. Their vitals are HR 122, BP 72/44, RR 32, CVP of 2, and SpO2 88% on 1.0 FiO2 via NRB. Which of the following RSI medications would be most appropriate for this patient?

    A. Provide Ketamine 100mg
    B. Administer Versed 5 mg
    C. Admin Etomidate 20 mg
    D. Succinylcholine 100mg

19. Potential hazards of positive-pressure mechanical ventilation include which of the following?

    A. cardiac tamponade, HTN, tension pneumothorax
    B. pneumothorax, subcutaneous emphysema, low BP
    C. decreased cardiac output and poor oxygenation
    D. subcutaneous emphysema and cardiac tamponade

20. A surgical airway is indicated in any patient

    A. with trismus and whom you cannot get chest rise and fall with BVM.
    B. with a large pharyngeal mass yielding 94% sats with rescue device.
    C. with massive facial fractures despite adequate SpO2 and EtCO2.
    D. with a tracheal surgical scar and who presents with COPD exacerbation.

21. As you are preparing to RSI your renal failure patient, you notice them to be breathing with pursed lips . Wheezes are present. Which of the following RSI regimens would be ideal?

    A. Versed, succinylcholine
    B. Ketamine, succinylcholine
    C. Etomidate, Zemuron
    D. Ketamine, rocuronium

22. You are preparing to RSI your patient and observe the following: HR 102, RR 26, BP 118/72, (+) peaked T waves on the 12 lead ECG. What is the ideal RSI regime?

    A. Versed, succinylcholine, rocuronium
    B. Ketamine, succinylcholine, pancurionium
    C. Etomidate, Fentanyl, zemuron,
    D. Morphine, Anectine, rocuronium

23. While pre-oxygenating a patient with BVM and positive end-expiratory pressure (PEEP), it is important to understand how PEEP works. Which of the following statements is TRUE regarding PEEP?

    A. It occurs at the beginning of a machine breath
    B. It decreases the functional residual capacity (FRC)
    C. It causes an increased venous return
    D. It may reduce minute ventilation (VE)

24. As you arrive at a rural ER, you find a 9 kg infant who has just experienced a return of spontaneous. CPR was performed for 4 minutes. You are currently preparing to RSI the infant. Which of the following partial RSI regimens is most appropriate?

A. 0.81 of Atropine, 10 mg of Rocuronium
B. 10 mg Ketamine, 18 mg Succinylcholine
C. 20 mg Succinylcholine, 20 mg Fentanyl
D. 0.2 mg of Versed, 18 mg of Rocuronium

25. Which of the following patients would a NPA be inappropriate to place?

A. 20 y/o with an unstable mid-face
B. 45 y/o with an identified C3 fracture
C. 25 y/o with a massive GI bleed
D. 32 y/o with severe bronchospasm

26. While caring for a patient who is mechanically ventilated and on positive end-expiratory pressure (PEEP). Which of the following statements is TRUE regarding PEEP?

A. It is applied during spontaneous inspiration involving SIMV
B. It increases the surface area of the alveolar membrane
C. It dramatically increases the patient's inspiratory

reserve

D. It causes an increased venous return and cardiac output

27. You find your trauma patient's dentures in the vehicle they just crashed. You decide to intubate the patient. Using this information, which of the following acronyms initially concerns you?

A. MOANS
B. RODS
C. LEMON
D. SHORT

28. Your patient has exceptionally thick facial hair. Which of the following acronym suggest caution when approaching this patient's airway?

A. SHORT
B. RODS
C. LEMON
D. MOANS

29. Choose the patient who most requires intubation.

A. Obtunded patient with a pH of 7.23
B. Heart attack patient with a 103 HR
C. COPD patient on a continuous nebulizer
D. SOB patient on BiPAP with 94% SPO2

30. You arrive at an ICU to retrieve a patient and you notice the ventilator on pressure control ventilation at 15/8 on 100% oxygen with normal I:E. This information tells you what about your patient?

A. The minute ventilation is 9 L
B. The I:E is measured at 1:4
C. Their PIP is 23 and PEEP is 8
D. The pressure control is 19

31. A 73 kg patient with altered mental status is intubated and has the following ventilator settings: A/C 16 VT 510 FIO2 100%, PEEP 5. His vital signs are BP 108/67 HR 88, SPO2 96%, ETCO2 49. The next most appropriate action is to?

A. TV 550
B. FiO2 0.7
C. RR 14
D. PEEP 7

32. Your patient's vital signs are BP 108/78, HR 101, O2 sats 94%, RR 22, and EtCO2 51. Which of the following is the best description of the patient's status?

A. Low oxygenation
B. Pre- hypotensive
C. Mild tachycardia
D. Poor ventilation

Answers

1. (**D**) the best sequence here should follow the sedative/ paralytic sequence and it should avoid anything that could drop BP. Versed drops BP. Answer choice B is incorrect because you need to administer a sedative before a paralytic. Therefore, D is the only option.

2. (**A**) This patient has an increased EtCO2 (52 mmHg) and to correct this problem we need to increase his minute ventilation. We could either increase RR or increase TV. There is no option to increase RR, but there is an option to increase TV, therefore, it is the correct answer.

3. (**C**) Preoxygenation is achieved by several means, including, but not limited to, BVM with a PEEP valve attached, passive oxygenation, sitting the head of the bed up at ~30 degrees, and attempt to achieve the sniffing position (tragus of ear aligned with the sternum) among others.

4. (**A**) The number one reason to execute a surgical airway is an inability to <u>intubate</u> AND an inability to <u>ventilate</u>. If you cannot "place the ETT" or cannot achieve good ventilations, then by definition you cannot intubate and cannot ventilate and a surgical airway is indicated.

5. (**B**) All of the dosing units or dosing are wrong on all the medications except Atropine- and the dosing is correct as well for atropine. Fentanyl 0.5-1 mcg/kg. Rocuronium 0.6-1.2 mg/kg. Ketamine 1-2 mg/kg.

6. (**B**) The combination of Fentanyl, Ketamine, Rocuronium is most appropriate in this case because all the answer options with succinylcholine are wrong as well as any answer with versed. All

the succinylcholine are wrong because the patient is bound to a wheelchair, so his lack of movement predisposes him to hyperkalemia following succinylcholine administration. All the versed answer options are incorrect because the patient has a MAP < 60 (MAP = 57 mmHg). Administering versed puts the patient at significant risk for hypotension.

7. (**A**) Rocuronium can be used on any patient. Fentanyl is great for pain control without reducing blood pressure much. Ketamine is a great medication for INCREASING blood pressure, however, it also bronchodilates the smaller airways. This feature makes answer A correct and the best benefit to this group of patients.

8. (**C**) While, yes, increasing the FiO2 will normally increase the SpO2, this case requires the ETT be backed up because it is too deep, right mainstemed, and thus has reduced minute ventilation (by about half) by only ventilating one lung. The only correct answer here is to back up the ETT. Remember, the appropriate depth is approximately 3 x ETT size. In this case, 7.0 x 3 = 21, therefore, the ETT is about 4 centimeters too deep- deep enough to go right main stem.

9. (**D**) The best sequence here should follow the sedative/ paralytic sequence and it should avoid anything that could drop BP. Ativan drops BP and sedatives must come before paralytics. Therefore, 'Ketamine, Anectine, zemuron' is the best option.

10. (**B**) This particular patient is absent a mental capacity to protect their airway (decreased LOC) and has no gag reflex (that normally protects the patient from aspiration). You need to secure the airway and an NPA/ OPA and suctioning will not secure the airway. An NPA or OPA, as well as BVM ventilations, would not be definitive. However, this patient needs their airway protected most of all, and thus is the correct answer (to intubate).Now, had this question asked what the "NEXT most

appropriate" then OPA would have been correct. "Next most appropriate" is specifically asking about the ORDER of treatment, whereas "most appropriate" typically is asking what is definitive. This is an item writer's (test question architect) trick, so commit this to memory.

11. (**B**) This particular patient is absent a mental capacity to protect their airway (decreased LOC) and has no gag reflex (that normally protects the patient from aspiration). You need to secure the airway and an NPA and suctioning will not secure the airway. A tracheostomy and ETT would do the job, so use the less invasive option: ETT, or endotracheal intubation.

12. (**A**) Every answer with versed is incorrect because the patient is showing signs of poor perfusion and a benzo could drop blood pressure. Answer C is the correct regimen, but A is the most correct because it is the right dosing and has the right dosing units.

13. (**C**) This is the only answer without succinylcholine (Anectine is the brand name of succinylcholine). This patient has been bedbound for several days and will be pre-disposed to hyperkalemia. This contraindicates succinylcholine.

14. (**C**) While, yes, increasing the FiO2 will normally increase the SpO2, this case requires the ETT be backed up because it is too deep, right mainstemed, and thus has reduced minute ventilation (by about half) from only ventilating one lung. The only correct answer here is to back up (or reposition) the ETT. The x-ray information, along with the low SpO2 and high EtCO2, indicate a right mainstemed ETT.

15. (**A**) Patient's with pulmonary embolism exhibit failure to oxygenate. Air has a way to get into the lungs, but cannot communicate with the blood, so a shunt occurs (air in and out does not match the blood going round and round).

16. (**C**) Succinylcholine is contraindicated in patients susceptible to hyperkalemia (like renal failure patients, patients who are bedbound, paraplegics/ quadriplegics, and any neuromuscular pathology). Therefore, the only patent here that is susceptible to hyperkalemia is the renal patient. They have kidney disease (therefore likely has higher potassium) and is poorly ambulatory (so they will be susceptible to hyperkalemia for this reason too). A new onset CVA with extremity weakness has not yet had time to develop the pathophysiology predisposing the patient to hyperkalemia from succinylcholine administration.

17. (**A**) Bronchospasm can be attenuated by ketamine, therefore, this is the best answer since the shark fin pattern indicates bronchospasm.

18. (**A**) Answer options B and C are both contraindicated. Versed could further drop blood pressure and etomidate is contraindicated in the septic patient. This leaves succinylcholine and ketamine. Between these 2 options, ketamine has a bigger benefit in that it can actually elevate blood pressure thus potentially improving their condition.

19. (**B**) Positive pressure ventilation (PPV) forces air into a lung that normally pulls air into itself with negative pressure. This is foreign to our physiology and thus can be detrimental if used incorrectly. Any increase in intrathoracic cavity, such as the increase that occurs with PPV, there is a reduction in venous return to the heart, thus reducing preload to the heart. This reduction in preload translates into lower cardiac output. PPV allows for increased oxygenation (with PEEP and FiO2), so that option is incorrect. It also will not inherently cause a cardiac tamponade, so that option is also incorrect. Widening pulse pressure is a sign of cardiac tamponade, and we just said that PPV doesn't cause this condition, it this answer is option too. PPV can cause a pneumothorax and if there is a disruption in the bronchial tree, subcutaneous emphysema can occur.

20. (**A**) The number 1 reason to execute a surgical airway is an inability to intubate AND an inability to ventilate. If you cannot "place the ETT" or cannot achieve a good tidal volume, then by definition you cannot intubate and cannot ventilate.

21. (**D**) Bronchospasm (breathing through pursed lips and wheezing) can be attenuated by ketamine, therefore, this is the best answer in this limited information question. Because the patient is a renal failure patient, succinylcholine should be avoided to prevent hyperkalemia.

22. (**C**) This is the only answer without succinylcholine (Anectine is the brand name of succinylcholine). This patient has peaked T-waves which suggests hyperkalemia, thus, contraindicates succinylcholine.

23. (**C**) If you increase PEEP beyond 8 cmH2o, you cause a tamponade effect and resulting poor forward blood flow though the lung vasculature. This causes blood to backup into the vena cava, jugular vein, and into the brain which can rise ICP. When increasing PEEP in the neuro patient, you will want to avoid increasing PEEP beyond 8 cmH2O. While the literature reports this as controversial, please still know the mechanism for the FPC, CCPC, and CFRN exams.

24. (**B**) All of the dosing is wrong on these medications except answer B. Atropine 0.02 mg/kg (max 1 mg, min 0.1 mg. Fentanyl 0.5-1 mcg/kg. Succinylcholine 1-2 mg/kg. Versed 2-4 mg. Rocuronium 0.6-1.2 mg/kg. Ketamine 1-2 mg/kg. The ketamine/ succinylcholine combination is the only correct dosing.

25. (**A**) NPAs are contraindicated when the patient has nasal fractures or basal skull fractures. An unstable mid-face is suggesting a La Fort fracture thus contraindicating NPAs.

26. (**B**) PEEP will cause 2 different therapeutic phenomenons: it will increase alveolar membrane surface area, and it will thin the

alveolar membrane. Both of these mechanisms will improve oxygenation. PEEP is very important during pre-oxygenation preparation.

27. (**A**) The dentures indicates that this patient could potentially be a difficult patient to ventilate (with BVM). With this in mind, it is important that you plan to have a backup plan and then back that plan up with a third backup plan. The point being: always be prepared and never let a situation catch you off guard. MOANS → difficult BVM ventilation; LEMON → difficult intubation; RODS → difficult rescue device placement; and SHORT → difficult cricothyrotomy.

28. (**D**) The beard indicates that this patient could potentially be a difficult patient to ventilate. With this in mind, it is important that you plan to have a backup plan and then back that plan up with a third backup plan. The point being: always be prepared and never let a situation catch you off guard. MOANS ⍰ difficult BVM ventilation; LEMON ⍰ difficult intubation; RODS ⍰ difficult rescue device placement; and SHORT ⍰ difficult cricothyrotomy.

29. (**A**) The heart attack patient is simply tachycardic and does not indicate intubation. The SOB patient does not indicate intubation either because they are maintaining their saturations. The COPD patient simply does not provide enough information for us to make a decision. The patient who does require intubation is the obtunded patient with a pH of 7.23 You could argue that they're expected clinical course could require intubation as well as failure to protect the airway as well as failure to auction it.

30. (**C**) The verbal shorthand "15/8" is telling you that the pressure control (PC) is set at 15 and the PEEP is set at 8. You add these numbers together to get 23, so the PIP is 23. The ventilator is set to deliver 15 cmH2O into the patients lungs which is on top of the 8 cmH2O of PEEP that was left over from the last breath

for a total of 23 cmH2O. Normal I:E is 1:2, so the I:E option is incorrect. We do not have the information to know the minute ventilation, so that option is also wrong. (More vent questions in respiratory!)

31. (**A**) This patient has an increased EtCO2 (52 mmHg) and to correct this problem we need to increase his minute ventilation. We could either increase RR or increase TV. There is no option to increase RR, but there is an option to increase TV, therefore, it is the correct answer. (More vent questions in respiratory!)

32. (**D**) Ventilatory status is identified by evaluating EtCO2, or if using an ABG then it is evaluated by the pCO2.

5 NEUROLOGY

Questions

---

1. A 56 y/o patient slipped in the bathroom, struck their head on the sink, and immediately lost consciousness. This was witnessed by a spouse. Upon your arrival, the patient is awake but then loses consciousness again right in front of you. Which condition does this describe?

   A. Autonomic dysreflexia
   B. Epidural hematoma
   C. Diffuse axonal injury
   D. Subdural hematoma

2. Upon responding to a patient with altered mental status who was a malnourished elderly patient, you note he only groans to painful stimuli and localizes the painful stimuli with his upper extremities. At the time of assessment, his blood sugar was 99 mg/dL and his pupils are 4mm and reactive bilaterally. V/S: BP 133/82, HR 99, RR 20, SpO2

95%. Which of the following treatments is most appropriate?

A. Thiamine
B. 1 amp D50
C. Calcium
D. Magnesium

3. TBI is the diagnosis of the patient currently in your care. It is an adult who suffered a rollover MVC. Which of the following is the best general treatment for this type of patient?

A. Keep the head of bed between 30-45°
B. Maintain O2 sats > 94% and MAP > 90
C. Target EtCO2 endpoint of 25-20 mmHg
D. Avoid the use of sedation and paralysis

4. As you are preparing to transport a patient with a cranial drain, you are calculating what your blood pressure minimal would need to be to maintain a 70 mmHg CPP. The patient's ICP monitor is showing 31 mmHg. What mean arterial pressure would you need to target to achieve this CPP?

A. 107
B. 102
C. 115
D. 101

5. You are transporting a patient who has a vetriculostomy and pressure monitoring. Which of the following is true regarding zeroing the pressure line?

    A. Align at the foramen of magnum
    B. Limit zeroing to the initial evaluation
    C. Set the head of the bed at 30-45°
    D. Avoid removing the transducer cap

6. You are calculating MAP on your head injury patient. Assume and ICP of 25mmHg. What is patient's CPP if your patient has a blood pressure of 135/75?

    A. 70
    B. 80
    C. 75
    D. 65

7. You are caring for a TBI patient. Which of the following vital sign values would make you confident that you were preventing secondary brain injury?

    A. BP 82/60, SpO2 90%, EtCO2 21
    B. BP 108/56, SpO2 91%, EtCO2 34
    C. BP 155/87, SpO2 96%, EtCO2 42
    D. BP 88/66, SpO2 99%, EtCO2 46

8. You ask an 88 y/o altered mental status patient what date it is and he says "yes, please." You note left-sided weakness when he grips your fingers, and looks at you when you speak to him. What is his Glasgow Coma Score.

   A. 11
   B. 13
   C. 12
   D. 14

9. You are treating a patient with a vetriculostomy drain and presents with high ICP. Which of the following is true with respect to management of this patient?

   A. No more than 3 cc of CSF should be removed at a time
   B. The CSF should not be drained if ICP is over 20 mmHg
   C. Measure and record the drain pressure every 2-3 hours
   D. Use normal saline with a bacteriostatic preservative

10. A 34 y/o motorcyclist suffered a crash and presents with mid-thoracic step off and a persistent erection. The patient's blood sugar is 130 mg/dL, both pupils are 4mm and briskly reactive to light and the patient can answer questions appropriately. V/S: BP 68/40, HR 101, RR 24, SpO2 86%. Which condition does this best describe?

    A. Subarachnoid hemorrhage
    B. Autonomic hypoflexia
    C. Traumatic brain injury
    D. Spinal cord injury

11. Your adult patient can obey simple commands and opens their eyes when they hear you speak. They can talk to you in sentences and seem a little confused and unsure of where they are. What is their current Glasgow Coma Scale score?

    A. 12
    B. 15
    C. 14
    D. 13

12. You are arriving at a small ER to retrieve a TBI patient. You notice the respiratory therapist is ventilating the patient at approximately 40 times per minute with an adult BVM. Which of the following dangerous pathophysiologies would this cause?

    A. Physiologic eucapnia
    B. Pathologic hypercapnia
    C. Systemic vasodilation
    D. Cerebral vasoconstriction

13. Your patient has an unstable mid-face to the degree that the maxilla, nasal, and portions of the zygoma all move when manually manipulated by grabbing the front teeth and pulling in an anterior (frontward) direction. Which Le Fort fracture is present?

A. I
B. II
C. III
D. IV

14. A 21 y/o mixed martial arts fighter is complaining of severe HA after a fight. His trainer reports that about 30 min after the fight, he became increasingly sleepy. After an hour after the fight, the trainer says he became unarousable. The patient's pupils are both dilated to ~ 8mm and poorly reactive to light. During the exam, the patient begins to posture. V/S: 198/ 104, HR 48, RR 28, SpO2 99%. Blood sugar is 104 mg/dL Which of the following conditions does this describe?

A. Ischemic stroke
B. Intracerebral hemorrhage
C. Wernicke's encephalopathy
D. Epidural hemorrhage

15. You're transporting an ICU patient with the following vital signs and findings: HR 62, BP 159/77, RR 26 and irregular, ICP monitor reads 23, CVP 17, and wedge pressure 15. Which the following is the most appropriate action?

A. Re-shoot a wedge pressure
B. Drain the vetriculostomy
C. Administer metoprolol
D. Prepare for cardiac arrest

16. A TBI patient is being transported from a small local hospital to a tertiary neurological center. Which of the following would best indicate increasing ICP?

    A. When the patient mentions a HA during ascent
    B. The patient complaining of acute severe nausea
    C. An increase of heart rate and a decrease of BP
    D. Noticing drowsiness and ipsilateral pupil changes

17. A motorcyclist suffers a crash an hits his head on the motorcycle handlebars. He complains of a small headache at the time and later that evening mentioned that his headache was still present, but 'not too bad.' The next morning, his wife reported he was slurring words and not answering questions (~ 15 hours s/p impact). At the time of EMS transport, his blood sugar was 84 mg/dL and his pupils were 4mm and sluggish bilaterally. V/S: BP 134/70, HR 72, RR 18, SpO2 99%.

    A. Subarachnoid injury
    B. Subdural hematoma
    C. Epidural hematoma
    D. Spinal cord injury

18. Your head injury patient with a cranial drain has an ICP of 22 mmHg. The patient's current blood pressure of 110/75. What is the most appropriate action in this case?

    A. Administer fluid boluses
    B. Immediately intubate
    C. Drain 3 cc of CSF fluid
    D. Place in Trendelenburg

19. A 35 y/o rollover MVC patient struck his head on the pavement upon ejection and was diagnosed with diffuse axonal injury. The sending physician states he was comatose for 28 hours but then regained consciousness and never postured. Which of these conditions does this describe?

    A. Diffuse axonal injury (severe)
    B. Diffuse axonal injury (progressive)
    C. Diffuse axonal injury (moderate)
    D. Diffuse axonal injury (mild)

20. An adult factory worker was on break speaking with a co-worker when he began to stare off into space and then began convulsing. The EMS report confirms a blood sugar of 88 mg/dL and pupils were at 4mm bilaterally and reactive to light. V/S: BP 130/70, HR 87, RR 18, SpO2 98%. Which condition matches this description?

    A. Tonic-clonic seizure
    B. Bacterial meningitis
    C. Severe hypoglycemia
    D. Autonomic dysreflexia

21. An adult boxer was struck several times during a match resulting in the referee calling the match. Following the match he complained of a severe HA and went to the ER. He initially exhibited an intact mental status, but began to become increasingly confused and later combative. She has no history and is on no medications. His pupils are 3 mm on the right and 6 mm on the left. V/S: 165/92, HR 45,

RR 23, SpO2 99%. Which of the following is causing this deterioration?

A. Diffuse axonal injury
B. Acute ischemic stroke
C. Intracranial pressure
D. Transit ischemic attack

22. You are transporting a patient with a head bleed. Which of the following findings would be consistent with Cushing's Reflex?

A. HR 51, BP 177/92, CVP 7, RR 26
B. BP 162/62, tachypnea, HR 99
C. RR 24, HR 75, hypotensive
D. Systolic BP 100, RR 16, HR 70

23. A 62 y/o female states she has a headache that began yesterday when she was moving furniture. Since then, she has had increasing eye pain and blurred vision. The only other symptom she has is some facial numbness. Her only history is a-fib. Vital signs are: BP 162/92, HR 52, SpO2 98%, RR 16. These symptoms are indicative of which of the following?

A. Wernicke encephalopathy
B. Diffuse axonal injury
C. Berry aneurysm
D. Subarachnoid hemorrhage

24. A 23 y/o male was attacked and struck multiple times with a crow bar. He complains of an inability to feel or move his lover extremities. He complains of HA, severe nausea. V/S: BP 162/108, HR 125, RR 26, SpO2 100%. Which of these conditions does this describe?

A. Autonomic dysreflexia
B. Epidural hematoma
C. Traumatic brain injury
D. Central cord syndrome

25. An ATV crash patient has multiple facial fractures. They have fractures to the maxilla, but the nasal bones and zygomas are intact. How would you classify this?

A. III
B. I
C. II
D. IV

Answers

1. (**B**) This patient presents with the classic signs of an epidural bleed. This classic presentation includes the patient losing consciousness, having a lucid period afterwards, and then returns to unconsciousness. In cases like these you should be highly suspicious of an epidural bleed. In this particular case, you witness the patient go from lucid to unconscious forming the unconscious-lucid-unconscious pattern consistent with epidural bleeds.

2. (**A**) Thiamine is the appropriate treatment. Wernicke's encephalopathy a condition where thiamine is deficient. Thiamine is important in facilitating glucose metabolism. Thiamine deficiencies are typically seen and people who do not take in enough vitamins, such as people who are malnourished. This is a common finding an alcoholics and homeless people.

3. (**B**) TBI patients should be managed generally by targeting O2 sats of 95% or greater and MAPs at 90 mmHg or greater. The head of the bed should be between 15-30°. EtCO2 should be targeted at 30-40, depending on the institution and literature (there seems to be a consensus at 35-40 mmHg currently). Sedation and paralysis are common place to keep the patient's ICP from increasing due to patient being awake and responding to the medical transport environment. The best answer here is "Maintain O2 sats > 94% and MAP > 90".

4. (**D**) This is a simple skill where we need to calculate MAP and CPP. To calculate MAP, double the diastolic pressure and add it to the systolic pressure. Take this value in divided by three. You have now arrived at your mean arterial pressure (MAP). To identify cerebral perfusion pressure (CPP) take your MAP and

subtract the total ICP. That value is your cerebral perfusion pressure (CPP). In this case, the CPP needs to be 70 mmHg. CPP = MAP - ICP, so set "x" for MAP. 70 (CPP) = X- 31 (ICP), this equals 70 + 31 = MAP, or 101 = MAP. If the patient has an ICP of 31 mmHg, then the MAP would need to be 101 mmHg to ensure a CPP of 70 mmHg.

5. (**C**) When transporting patients with pressure lines, zeroing is important. Align the transducer at the foramen of Monroe, re-zero with each patient move and with ascent and decent, sit the patient's HOB to 30-45°, and be sure to remove the cap when zeroing the line.

6. (**A**) This is a simple skill where we need to calculate MAP and CPP. To calculate MAP, double the diastolic pressure and add it to the systolic pressure. Take this value in divided by three. You have now arrived at your mean arterial pressure (MAP). To identify cerebral perfusion pressure (CPP) take your MAP and subtract the total ICP. That value is your cerebral perfusion pressure (CPP). MAP is calculated at 95 mmHg in this case. MAP - ICP in this case is 70.

7. (**C**) There are two answers with hypoxia: 90% and 91%, which can cause secondary brain injury. Therefore these answer selections are incorrect. There are two true hypotensive blood pressures: 82 and 88 systolic, therefore this could cause secondary brain injury. These are also incorrect answer selections. The only correct answer suggesting secondary brain injury prevention: BP 155/87, SpO2 96%, EtCO2 42.

8. (**B**) The patient and looks at you earns a GCS eye opening score of 4. A patient who answers questions inappropriately earns them a GCS verbal score of 3. In this case, your patient is gripping your fingers, therefore she is following commands. Following commands gets you a GCS motor score of 6. E4 + V3 + M6 = GCS of 13.

9. (**A**) When managing a patient with a vetriculostomy drain, never remove more than 3 cc of CSF at a time, only drain per MD orders or when the ICP is OVER 20 mmHg, measure and record pressure every hour, and never use a NS with a bacteriostatic preservative in the pressure bag of the drain set up.

10. (**D**) There are three things that indicate spinal cord injury in this case. The patient's priapism- damage to a male's spinal cord prevents the muscle that keeps blood out of penis from remaining constricted. Once it is relaxed from SCI, the penis is allowed to fill with blood. Hypotension occurs because the spinal cord injury (SCI) also relaxes the smooth muscle in vessels. Once they relax, vasodilation occurs and hypotension follows. Subarachnoid hemorrhage and traumatic brain injury both present with altered mental status typically, it doesn't fit the profile here. Autonomic hyporeflexia is not a real condition. Ever choose the answer that you are unfamiliar with- Ever.

11. (**D**) This patient does not open their eyes spontaneously, but when you call their name. This earns them a GCS eye opening score of 3. If your patient answered questions, then they are following commands and earns than a GCS motor score of 6. The fact that they are confused indicates there verbal score is 4. E3 + V4 + M6 = GCS of 13.

12. (**D**) This patient is currently being hyperventilated, therefore their carbon dioxide measurements will be low. This causes a vasoconstriction within the cerebral blood flow. This is dangerous because it limits the blood flow to the delicate and sensitive brain tissue. It is important to only hyperventilate with signs of brain herniation, and still only targeting carbon dioxide levels between 30 and 40 mmHg- depending on current literature.

13. (**C**) In this case we have complete craniofacial separation, therefore this is a Le fort III. Le Fort fractures are fractures of

the midface, which collectively involve separation of all or a portion of the midface from the skull base. Le Fort type 1: [horizontal maxillary fracture, separating the teeth from the upper face, fracture line passes through the alveolar ridge, lateral nose and inferior wall of maxillary sinus]; Le Fort type 2 [pyramidal fracture, with the teeth at the pyramid base, and nasofrontal suture at its apex, fracture arch passes through posterior alveolar ridge, lateral walls of maxillary sinuses, inferior orbital rim and nasal bones]; Le Fort type 3 [craniofacial disjunction, fracture line passes through nasofrontal suture, maxillo-frontal suture, orbital wall and zygomatic arch].

14. (**B**) A quick development of HA an, sleepiness, and altered level of consciousness indicates an epidural bleed. Additionally, you can see Cushing's reflex occurring (high BP, low HR) which indicates increasing ICP.

15. (**B**) The patient ICP has elevated beyond 20 mmHg, therefore it is important to drain the vetriculostomy to prevent herniation and symptomologies of increased ICP.

16. (**D**) This patient has recently received a traumatic brain injury, therefore it is important to look for signs of decreasing level of consciousness, posturing, and pupillary changes. Ipsilateral pupil changes and drowsiness is the most suggestive of increasing ICP in this case.

17. (**B**) This patient received a traumatic blow to the frontal skull that resulted in a small headache. The next morning he presented with stroke like symptoms. Subdural hematomas typically arise from veins, so they have a slow progression (which matches the 15 hours from impact to current symptoms) after some impact to the head. However they also can occur spontaneously. Epidurals happen usually rapidly because they

arise from arteries. Spinal cord injuries result in motor and sensory problems which is not present in this question, therefore the spinal cord injury option is incorrect.

18. (**C**) The patient is presenting with > 20 mmHg of ICP, and you may need to drain off some CSF. It is good practice to not drain out more than 3 cc at a time.

19. (**C**) Diffuse axonal injuries (DAIs) have three magnitudes: mild, moderate, and severe. Moderate DAI is indicated with comas lasting > 24 hours, no posturing noted, and a normal head CT. This is the correct answer in this case.

20. (**A**) The convulsing represents a tonic, or tonic-clonic type seizure. You can have seizures with hypoglycemia, but since the blood sugar is normal the hypoglycemia selection can be ruled out.

21. (**C**) This patient has a history of a direct blow to the head and a declining mental status. Additionally one pupil is enlarging indicating herniation. The symptom of increasing confusion is most likely due to an increased intracranial pressure (ICP).

22. (**A**) There is one answer here with a high blood pressure and bradycardia, which demonstrates Cushing's Reflex, therefore it is the answer. Cushing's reflex can be identified by a very high blood pressure (with widening pulse pressure) that occurs with bradycardia. This is the result of two different physiological systems working against one another. As a patient develops increasing ICP, the body will increase blood pressure in an effort to force open vessels in the brain. This increase in blood pressure acts as a fluid scaffolding to keep the vessels opened against the increasing pressure. The heart recognizes the increase in blood pressure, and thinks it's a bad thing. So the heart slows down to reduce blood pressure. Therefore we get an increasing blood pressure in a decreasing heart rate. You also

can have increased respiratory rates and irregular respiratory patterns, but it is more from the increasing the ICP rather than the blood pressure/ heart rate war.

23. (**C**) Aneurysms occur via a weakening in the arterial wall of a vessel in the brain which eventually ruptures. This can lead to headache, eye pain and visual changes, numbness in weakness, altered level of consciousness as well as increasing ICP. Autonomic dysreflexia and diffuse axonal injury typically requires a traumatic event. Wernicke's encephalopathy is from a thiamine deficiency. The best answer in this case is berry aneurysm. Even if you don't know the specific type of aneurysm, these are the signs and symptoms of an aneurysm.

24. (**A**) This patient has had obvious damage to his spinal cord resulting in a strange reaction by the autonomic nervous system where blood pressure increases, heart rate increases, as well as nausea and vomiting. This is called autonomic dysreflexia.

25. (**B**) The orbital bones, the nasal bones and the maxilla bones are all intact. This is a Le Fort I injury.

6 CARDIOLOGY

Questions

1. The critical care transport clinician is caring for a patient receiving a continuous norepinephrine (Levophed) infusion. Which of the following information indicates that the infusion is not effective, and that a second pressor may be warranted?

   A. CO
   B. PCWP
   C. SVR
   D. CVP

2. Examine the following IABP tracing, then choose the appropriate assessment of this tracing.

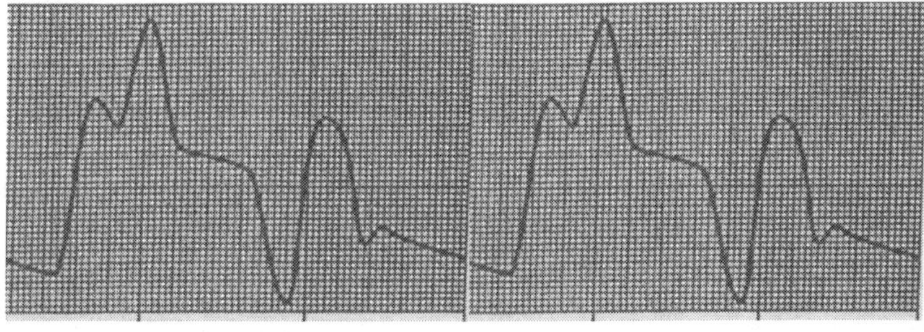

A. Early inflation
B. Late inflation
C. Early deflation
D. Late deflation

3. Which of the following hemodynamic values are within their normal limits?

A. SVR of 120
B. PCWP 25
C. CVP of 4
D. CO of 12

4. Upon evaluating the patient's hemodynamic parameters, you note an SVR of 1800. Which of the following is the best general treatment plan?

A. Administer beta blockers
B. Administer isotonic fluids
C. Administer a vasopressor
D. Administer a vasodilator

5. Upon assessment of your cardiac patient, you notice p-waves on the 12 lead that are tall and pointy. This is caused by which of the following:

A. Increased cardiac output
B. High right atrial pressures
C. Massive hyperkalemia
D. Reduced SVR and CVP

6. When assessing your cardiac patient, you assess heart tones. You recall the S1 sound is equivalent to which of the following:

   A. Isovolumetric relaxation
   B. Closure of the AV valve
   C. The P wave on the ECG
   D. The aortic valve opening

7. You are assessing a 12 lead ECG. You identify the following: PR interval of 80 milliseconds, QRS < 100 milliseconds, and a Q wave that is half the height of the R wave. Which of the following is most likely present?

   A. Hypothermia present
   B. Pathological Q waves
   C. Anterioseptal AMI
   D. WPW syndrome

8. You have a patient with a wide QRS waveform (150ms). A retrograde (reverse direction) upward deflection from the J point in V1 on a 12 lead ECG. Which of the following is present?

   A. Left bundle branch block
   B. Present left axis deviation
   C. Right bundle branch block
   D. Present right axis deviation

9. You are assessing for an AMI in your patient. You notice in V6 ST elevation of 2 mm in height with a positive QRS, and ST depression in V3 of 3 mm with a negative QRS complex. How many points does this earn when the Sgarbossa criteria is applied?

    A. 2 points
    B. 4 points
    C. 6 points
    D. 8 points

10. Upon evaluating a 12 lead on your cardiac patient, you notice P pulmonale and biphasic P wave in V1. Which of the following does this indicate?

    A. This is a normal finding
    B. Left Atrial enlargement
    C. Right Atrial enlargement
    D. A biatrial enlargement

11. You are assessing a cardiac patient and notice in V2 a S wave and in V6 a R wave added together is 37 mm. What does this indicate?

    A. Left ventricular hypertrophy
    B. Right ventricular hypertrophy
    C. Left atrial hypertrophy
    D. Right atrial hypertrophy

12. Preload, afterload and contractility are all components that can influence which of the following?

    A. The amount of blood ejected by the heart per beat
    B. The amount of blood ejected by the heart per minute
    C. Pressures experienced by the pulmonary artery
    D. Increasing right and left ventricular systolic pressures

13. Upon assessing a 12 lead of your cardiac patient being transferred for cath lab, you note ST-elevation in V1, V2 and slightly in V3. Which coronary artery feeds this location of the heart?

    A. Left coronary artery
    B. Right coronary artery
    C. Anterior coronary artery
    D. Posterior coronary artery

14. Examine the following hemodynamic pressure monitor tracing, then choose the appropriate assessment of this tracing.

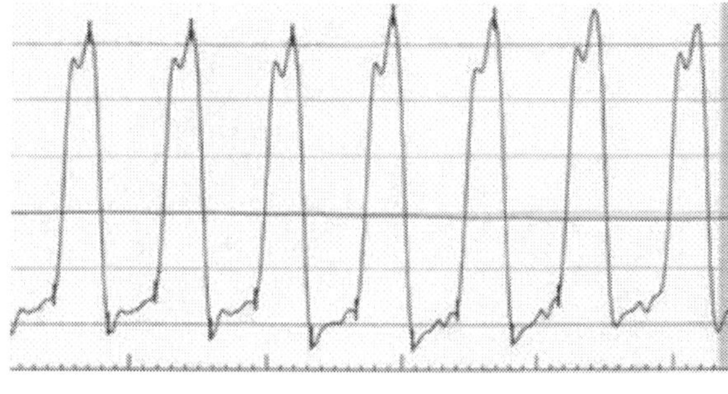

A. LV is throwing runs of ventricular tach
B. A superwedge is currently progressing
C. PA catheter has migrated to the RV
D. A retrograde PA cath movement

15. On assessment of a chest x-ray, you notice a heart silhouette that is half the size of the chest itself and has very rounded edges (looks circular). What kind of treatment is required?

    A. Palliative care only
    B. Copious fluid resuscitation
    C. Vasopressors are a must
    D. Same as with heart failure

16. Your 67 y/o cardiac/ chest pain patient presents with ST segment elevation, no hyperacute T waves and no pathological Q waves. Which phase of AMI progression is the patient currently in?

    A. Acute phase I
    B. Acute phase II
    C. Hyperacute T waves
    D. Age indeterminate

17. Your patient currently presents with the following: HR 99, SpO2 87, BP 128/92, CVP 15, PCWP 10, CO 4, and 850 for SVR. Which of the following would you most likely assess in this patient?

A. Wet system
B. Vasopressors
C. PA cath in RA
D. Dehydration

18. Your 42 y/o chest pain patient has the following 12 lead findings: ST elevation in V5, V6, and lead I. Which coronary artery is most likely occluded?

A. Left anterior descending
B. Right coronary artery
C. Right circumflex artery
D. Left circumflex artery

19. Upon assessment of a 75 y/o male, you note a wide mediastinum and different blood pressures between their 2 arms. You recall the treatment for the condition this describes as

A. Keep BP >120mmHg systolic, negative inotropes first THEN vasodilators if needed
B. Keep BP <120mmHg systolic, vasodilators first THEN negative inotropes if needed
C. Keep BP <120mmHg systolic, negative inotropes first THEN vasodilators if needed
D. Keep BP >120mmHg systolic, vasodilators first THEN negative inotropes if needed

20. What physiologic changes would you expect following the administration of Levophed?

    A. Reduced vasoconstriction and HR
    B. Increased HR and blood pressure
    C. Elevated HR and vasodilation
    D. Reduced BP and increased HR

21. Your patient began having shortness of breath and chest pain over the last 2 hours. The patient reports that he is a CHF patient for 10 years with multiple stents placed in his heart, he has a dual pacer, and has been hospitalized twice in the last decade for his cardiac conditions. Examine the ECG tracing below. Which of the following is the patient most likely experiencing?

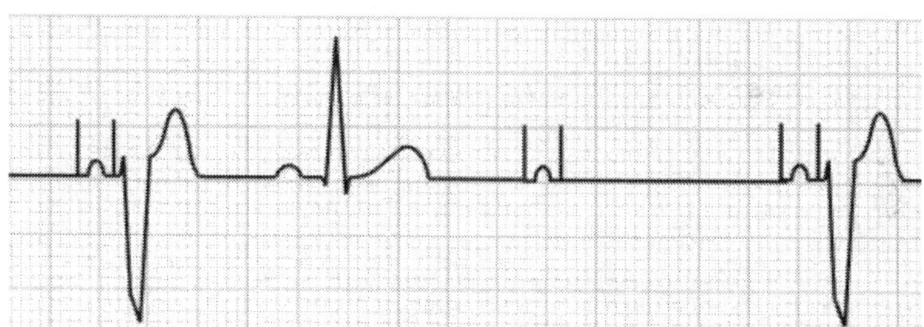

    A. There is a left bundle branch block present
    B. Failure of the ventricular pole to capture
    C. Hypoxia is present and will soon exacerbate
    D. The pointy P waves indicate p- pulmonale

22. You are transporting a 53 y/o on an IABP support. Which of the following would indicate the goals of IABP treatment are being met?

A. SVR 700
B. PCWP 5
C. CVP 12
D. CO of 6

23. Your adult cardiac patient has a pulmonary artery in place. You receive the following information: BP 92/52 mmHg, CO 2.8 L/min, and the PA temperature is 37 degrees C. Which of the following is dangerous?

A. PA temperature
B. Blood pressure
C. Cardiac output
D. All are normal

24. You are transporting an ICU to ICU patient and they present with the following vital signs: CVP 10, PCWP 14, CO 3, and 1050 for SVR. Which of the following medications would best treat this patient?

A. Nitroglycerine
B. LMW Heparin
C. Metoprolol
D. Integrillin

25. Which of the following patients appear hemodynamically compromised?

A. 67 y/o cardiac patient with CO 4.9 L/min
B. 8 m/o infant with cardiac output of 1 L/min
C. 5 y/o asthmatic patient with CO 2.0 L/min
D. 19 y/o trauma patient with CO 3.5 L/min

26. You are explaining to a new hire the significance of finding QRS notching and ST elevation on a 12 lead ECG. Which of the following assessments is most likely correct?

    A. Pericarditis likely is present
    B. Pericarditis likely is absent
    C. AMI is most likely present
    D. AMI is most likely absent

27. Your 24 y/o patient is experiencing sudden onset of shortness of breath. You observe the following findings: HR 92, BP102/70, SpO2 88%, an S wave in V1 of 10mm and R wave in V1 of 20 mm. Which of the following condition is most likely present?

    A. Status asthmaticus
    B. Myocardial infarction
    C. Congestive heart failure
    D. Pulmonary embolism

28. Examine the following IABP tracing, then choose the appropriate assessment of this tracing.

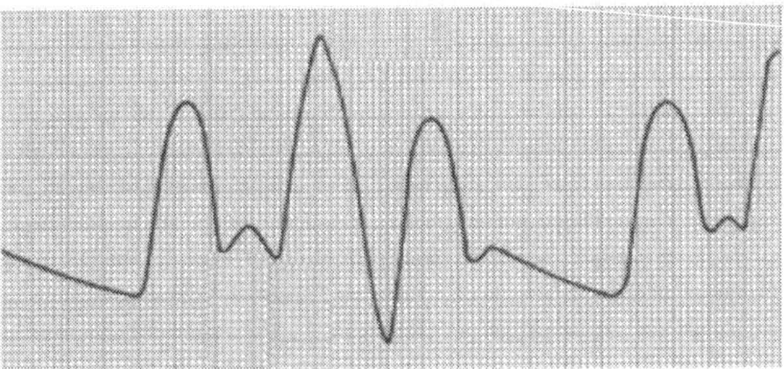

A. Early inflation
B. Late inflation
C. Early deflation
D. Late deflation

29. A patient presents to the ER after a few days after open heart surgery with a fever, malaise and shortness of breath. The patient has the following vitals and findings: HR 105, SpO2 98, BP 125/78, CVP 5, PCWP 5, CO 12, and 600 for SVR. What type of shock is this patient most likely exhibiting?

A. Distributive
B. Neurogenic
C. Septic shock
D. Cardiogenic

30. You are transporting a chest pain patient. The 55 y/o male's 12 lead shows elevation of the J point in the inferior leads. Which coronary artery is being blocked?

A. Left coronary artery
B. Right coronary artery
C. Anterior coronary artery
D. Posterior coronary artery

31. You are about to administer Levophed to a patient. What physiological changes would you anticipate following the administration of such a medication?

    A. Vasoconstriction and increasing HR
    B. Lowing blood pressure and tachycardia
    C. Increased BP and slower AV conduction
    D. Bronchoconstriction with bradycardia

32. While assessing your cardiac patient, you notice a ladle-like morphology. Because of this, your patient is most likely suffering which of the following?

    A. Hyperkalemia
    B. Digitalis toxicity
    C. Hypokalemia
    D. Mag toxicity

33. Hemodynamically, what do you expect Neosynepherine to do to your patient's hemodynamic parameters?

    A. ↓ PVR
    B. ↑CVP
    C. ↓ CO
    D. ↑ SVR

34. A patient with shortness of breath and chest pain exhibits an unique morphology of the QRS waveform in V1. Which of the following indicates a bundle branch block?

A. ST depression in leads I, II, and aVL
B. A short and flat hyper acute T wave
C. Presence of extreme right axis deviation
D. QRS complex spanning 4 small boxes

35. Examine these fishbone labs and identify the value that is out of range.

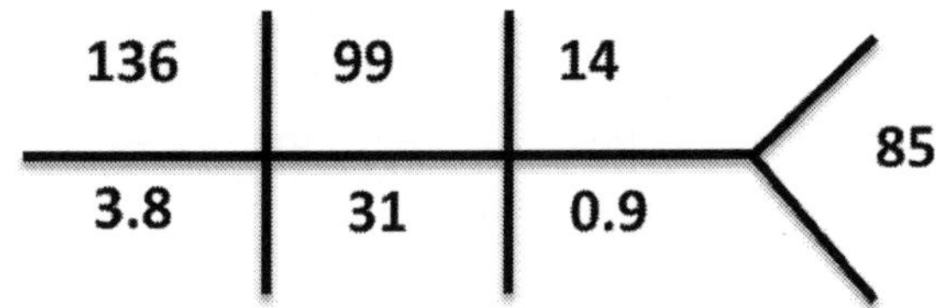

A. The glucose
B. Bicarbonate
C. The chloride
D. Potassium

36. Your patient has a PR segment below the isoelectric line and ST elevation in 10 of the 12 leads, including Lead I and II. Which of the following is the patient most likely experiencing?

A. Anterior AMI
B. Massive AMI
C. Pericarditis
D. Hyperkalemia

37. Your adult patient develops a HR of 44. You understand that this heart rate will result in which of the following?

    A. CO is reduced
    B. CO is elevated
    C. SV is reduced
    D. SV is elevated

38. While transporting a patient on IABP support, you notice a 'double V' pattern. This timing pattern characterizes which of the following?

    A. Early deflation
    B. Late deflation
    C. Early inflation
    D. Late inflation

39. During a transport of a patient with ST elevation in leads II, III, and aVF, you are considering initial pharmacological therapy. Which of the following constitute the best pharmacological choices?

    A. Aspirin, nitro, heparin, warfarin
    B. Aspirin, fluid bolus, nitro, oxygen
    C. Oxygen, beta blockers, versed
    D. Nitro, high molecular weight heparin

40. A 44 y/o male is being assessed for cardiac issues. You do not observe any ST elevation. Instead you see a large, deep Q wave. Their troponin is 4. Which phase of AMI progression is the patient currently in?

A. Acute phase I
B. Acute phase II
C. Hyperacute T waves
D. Age indeterminate

41. Your new hire hands you a 12 lead of your patient (+ ST-elevation in I, aVL, V5, and V6). You recall this is due to a blocked

A. Left anterior decending
B. Right coronary artery
C. Anterior coronary artery
D. Posterior coronary artery

42. You receive a report from the sending RN where they mention a specific condition characterized by serum being forced into the alveoli from back pressure of cardiac origin. This produces a foamy liquid which prevents adequate ventilation and oxygenation. Upon assessment, the patient has no JVD or acietes. Which of the following best identifies this pathophysiology?

A. Left sided heart failure
B. Right sided heart failure
C. Congestive heart failure
D. Chronic heart failure

43. A patient's vital signs are pulse 105, respirations 24, and BP of 112/70 mm Hg and cardiac output is 5.4 L/min. What is the patient's stroke volume?

    A. 61 mL
    B. 41 mL
    C. 51 mL
    D. 71 Ml

44. Which of the following hemodynamic values are within their normal limits?

    A. PCWP 11
    B. CVP of 10
    C. SVR of 80
    D. CO of 10

45. Your 55 y/o cardiac patient complaining of chest pain currently presents with a left bundle branch block on the 12 lead. What diagnostic tool could be used to confirm if an AMI is actually happening?

    A. Osborne waves in V1
    B. S to R Wave Ratio
    C. Hyperacute T waves
    D. Sgarbossa criteria

46. Examine these fishbone labs and identify the value that is out of range.

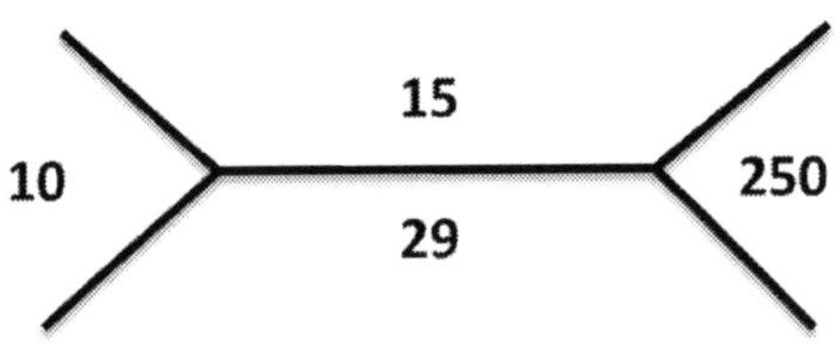

A. Platelets
B. The WBCs
C. Hematocrit
D. Hemoglobin

47. As you assess your ICU patient, you observe the following: HR 111, SpO2 84, BP 80/56, CVP 2, PCWP 5, CO 3, and 1650 for SVR. What type of shock is this patient exhibiting?

A. Septic shock
B. Distributive
C. Hypovolemic
D. Cardiogenic

48. You are transporting a patient from a cardiac floor to a cardiac specialty facility. Which of the following indicates left ventricular failure?

A. PA diastolic pressure 11
B. Stroke volume of 60cc
C. Wedge pressure of 16
D. Current CVP pressure of 5

49. As blood flow though the heart continues, pressure changes occur. Once there is greater pressure in the aorta and pulmonary artery, the semilunar valves close. Which of the following sounds does this closure represent?

    A. S1
    B. S2
    C. S4
    D. S3

50. Your 66 y/o chest pain patient has the following 12 lead findings: ST elevation in V1 and V2. Which coronary artery is most likely occluded?

    A. Left coronary artery
    B. The circumflex artery
    C. Left anterior descending
    D. Right coronary artery

51. While assessing a patient with tachycardia, you note a shortened PR and lengthened QRS. This makes the QRS appear somewhat triangular? Which of the following conditions would most likely be the cause?

    A. Acute pericarditis
    B. WPW syndrome
    C. Hyperkalemia
    D. Mag toxicity

52. Your patient has a T-wave 2/3 the height of the QRS complex in Lead II. They are pointed and not rounded. With this 12- lead feature, what would you most likely expect to find with this patient?

A. Digitalis level 2.1
B. This is normal
C. Potassium of 6.1
D. Calcium of 15.3

53. Examine the following IABP tracing, then choose the appropriate assessment of this tracing.

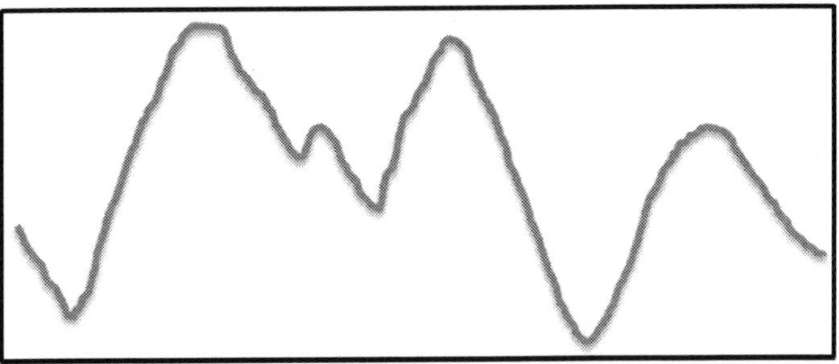

A. Early inflation
B. Late inflation
C. Early deflation
D. Late deflation

54. Your patient is exhibiting reduced heart sounds, engorged jugular veins, and shortness of breath and the MD mentions needing to perform a pericardiocentesis. You recall that the two common causes of the precipitating condition is which of the following?

A. Pericarditis and chest trauma
B. Chest trauma and pneumonia
C. Pneumonia and cardiogenic shock
D. Pericarditis and cardiogenic shock

55. Your patient presents with the following vitals and lab findings: BP 152/98, SpO2 96, CVP 5, PCWP 7, CO 7, and 1500 for SVR. Which of these parameters is MOST concerning?

A. PCWP 12
B. SVR 1500
C. CVP of 4
D. SpO2 95

56. You are transporting a chest pain patient who has an upright deflection in aVF and a downward deflection in Lead I. With this information, you know that there is also most likely which if the following?

A. Myocardial ischemia
B. Left anterior hemiblock
C. First degree heart block
D. Myocardial injury

57. Your 57 y/o chest pain patient has the following 12 lead findings: ST depression in V8 and V9, with ST elevation in V3 and V4. Which coronary artery is most likely occluded?

A. The circumflex artery
B. Right coronary artery
C. Left coronary artery
D. Left anterior descending

58. A 56 y/o chest pain patient is being transported to a tertiary facility. Upon assessment, you are considering left ventricular hypertrophy. You are assessing a QRS complex for left ventricular hypertrophy. Which of the following would indicate LVH is present?

A. aVR R wave is 10 mm
B. aVR S wave is 11 mm
C. aVL R wave is 12 mm
D. aVL S wave is 15 mm

59. A student asks you to summarize what happens in cardiogenic shock. Which of the following would best answer the student's question?

A. weakened pump, cardiac tamponade, global acidosis
B. weakened arterial walls, poor tissue perfusion, dysrhythmias
C. weakened arterial walls, cardiac tamponade, global edema
D. weakened pump, poor tissue perfusion, global acidosis

60. During the patient assessment, you notice the distal tip of your ICU patient's IABP balloon is observed at the 3rd intercostal space on x-ray. The critical care transport clinician understands that:

    A. This positioning is too low
    B. This positioning is too high
    C. The position is close enough
    D. The position is appropriate

61. Examine the following IABP tracing, then choose the appropriate assessment of this tracing.

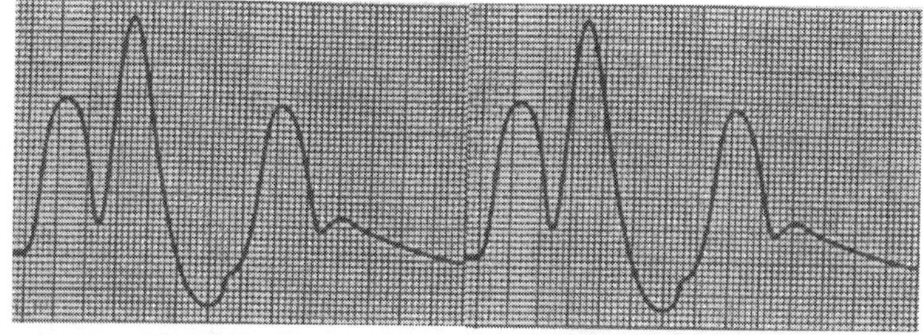

    A. Early inflation
    B. Late inflation
    C. Early deflation
    D. Late deflation

62. A 39 y/o male chest pain patient presents with following 12 lead findings: ST elevation in II, III and aVF; as well as ST depression in I and aVL. Which coronary artery is most likely occluded?

A. Left coronary artery
B. Right coronary artery
C. Right circumflex
D. Left circumflex artery

63. While transporting a septic patient, you note their central venous pressure (CVP) is 2mmHg. Which of the following is the most appropriate action?

A. Increase the IV fluids
B. Administer a pressor
C. Begin a nitro infusion
D. Limit vasopressor use

64. During an Interfacility transport, you note the following hemodynamic parameters on your patient's chart: CVP 12, PCWP 17, CO 3, and 1100 for SVR. What type of shock is this patient exhibiting?

A. Septic shock
B. Cardiogenic
C. Anaphylactic
D. Neurogenic

65. Hemodynamically, what do you expect the middle dosages (beta of dopamine to do to your patient's hemodynamic parameters?

A. ↓ PVR
B. ↑ PCWP
C. ↑ SVR
D. ↓ CO

66. A patient suffered a critical fall and has step off at the level of T-3 resulting in a demarcation at the level of the xyphoid process (red skin below this level). Which of the following treatments should this patient likely receive?

    A. Avoid administering vasopressors in this case
    B. Provide epi to achieve vasodilatory response
    C. Administer volume and then increase the SVR
    D. Deliver fluid boluses only- no vasopressor

67. Which of the following hemodynamic values are within their normal limits?

    A. Systolic RVP 19
    B. Diastolic PAP 9
    C. Diastolic RVP 19
    D. Systolic PAP 9

68. A new hire inquies about a cardiac condition caused by injury to the heart resulting in fluid accumulation encircling the pericardium which results in increasingly worsening cardiac output. What condition is this blog describing?

A. Congestive heart failure
B. Cardiomyopathy
C. Cardiogenic shock
D. Cardiac Tamponade

69. Your cardiac patient currently has the following ECG findings: lead I, lead III, and aVL is positive; lead II is isoelectric; and aVF and aVR is negative. Which of the following conditions is the patient most likely suffering from?

A. Anterioseptal AMI
B. Left axis deviation
C. Aortic Dissection
D. Coronary artery block

70. Which of the following hemodynamic values are within their normal limits?

A. Diastolic PAP 15
B. Diastolic RVP 10
C. Systolic PAP 10
D. Systolic RVP 30

71. A cardiac patient presents with a p wave in lead II with 2 'humps', no ST-elevation, and a QRS that is < 120 milliseconds. Which of the following is most likely the current condition?

A. Silent AMI is occurring
B. Right atrial enlargement
C. Diseased tricuspid valve
D. P mitrale is progressing

72. You are transporting a VAD patent. While conducting a routine assessment, you note that the patient doesn't have a pulse at any pulse site. The patient is calm, awake, and answering all questions. What kind of VAD does the patient have?

A. Pneumatic Flow
B. Asynchronous Flow
C. Continuous Flow
D. Pulsatile Flow

73. You are treating a patient involved in a MVC with massive external damage. The patient is a VAD patient and currently presents with the following: awake and alert, in pain, open clear airway, with a HR of 0, BP of 0, RR 22/min, SpO2 91%, EtCO2 44, skin cool and pink, with good capillary refill (< 2 seconds), however ventricular fibrillation is on the monitor. What is the next most appropriate action?

A. Supportive care
B. Defibrillation
C. Cardioversion
D. Precordial Thumb

74. Look at the below 12- lead and identify which wall of the myocardium is affected.

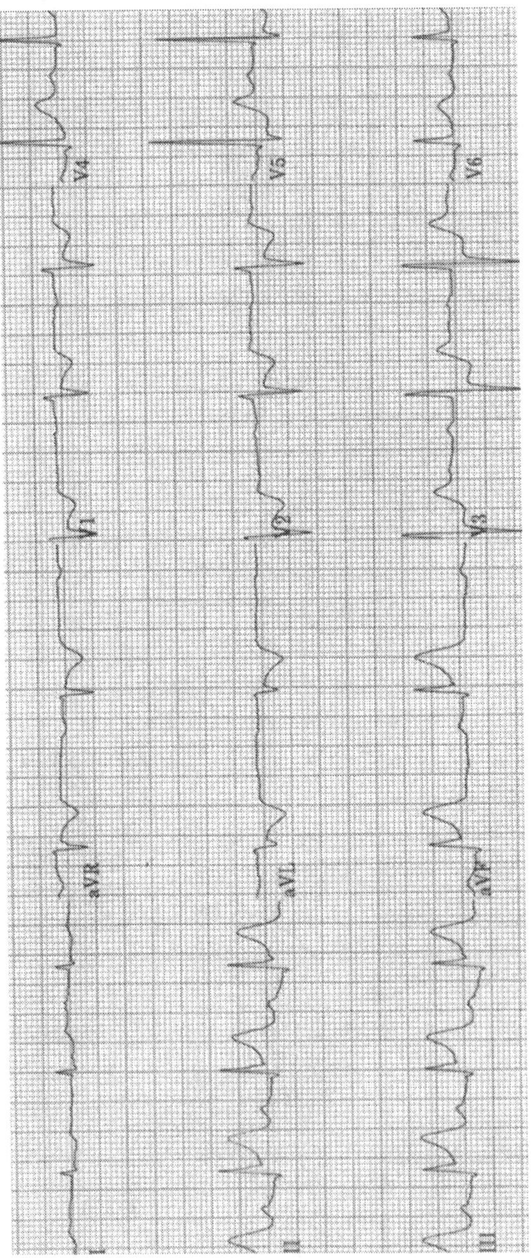

A. Lateral wall AMI
B. Anterior wall AMI
C. Inferior wall AMI
D. Septal wall AMI

75. Look at the below 12- lead and identify which wall of the myocardium is affected.

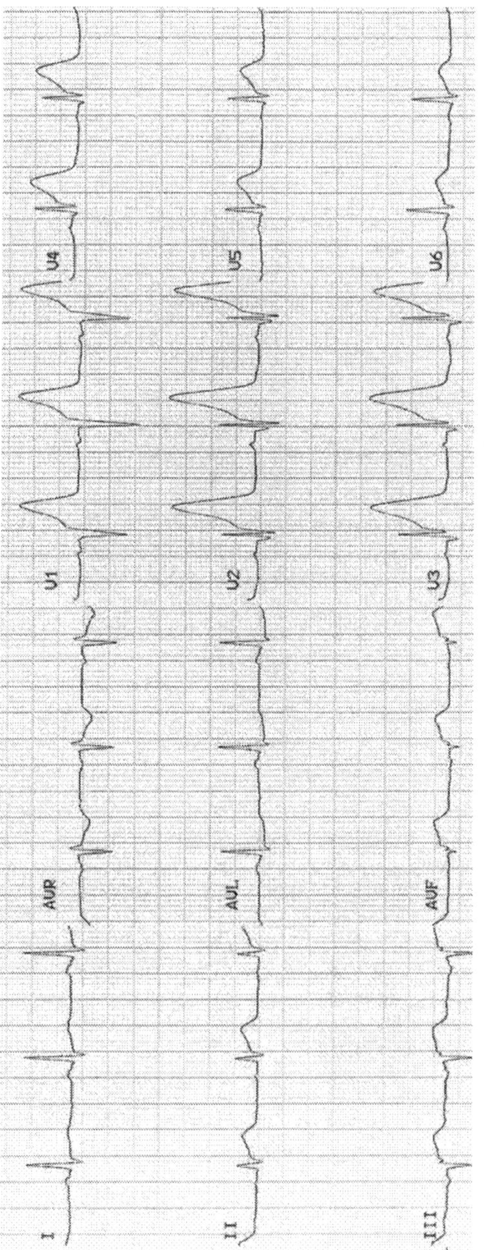

A. Inferiolateral wall AMI
B. High lateral wall AMI
C. Anterioseptal wall AMI
D. Inferioseptal wall AMI

76. Look at the below 12- lead and identify which wall of the myocardium is affected.

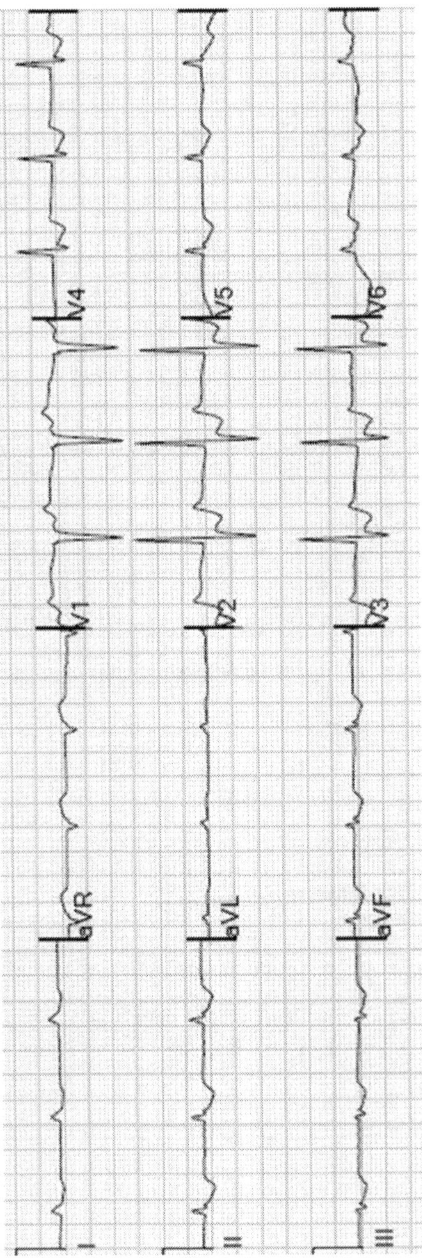

A. Inferiolateral wall AMI
B. Inferior wall AMI
C. Anterioseptal wall AMI
D. Posterior wall AMI

Answers

1. (**C**) Levophed increases alpha 1 stimulation (therefore increases SVR), which increases blood pressure. If you monitored SVR and it got very high without correcting blood pressure, then a new pressor may need to be added.

2. (**A**) Note a VERY high inflation point. First remember where the dicrotic notch should be. Now, look at this one. It is very high to the peak of the systole, most likely way before the dicrotic notch. This causes a lot of pressure against the compressing ventricles. This is the MOST DANGEROUS timing error.

3. (**C**) Normally, CVP is 2-8 mmHg, SVR is 800-1300 dynes/sec/cm^3, PCWP is 4-12 mmHg, and CO is normally 4-8 L/min. therefore, the only one in its normal range in this case is the CVP of 4.

4. (**D**) To answer this question, you need to know what afterload is and what treatments affect it. Afterload represents the pressure the heart has to pump against to eject blood into the aorta (left ventricle) and lungs (right ventricle). It is measured as the SVR (systemic vascular resistance). If SVR is normal, then there isn't too much pressure the heart has to pump against. If it is low, then it is very easy for the ventricles to pump blood. If it is high, then there is an awful lot of pressure the ventricles have to overcome in order to pump blood. Medications like vasodilators will dilate the arterial system, and thus reduce the SVR- which is the answer. Administering Vasopressors will increase SVR- bad. Adding fluid could also worsen this issue. Beta blockers would reduce cardiac output, but won't directly affect the afterload. The best choice here is to administer a vasodilator to reduce SVR and thus making it easier for the heart to pump (which also directly decreases myocardial oxygen demand).

5. (**B**) Tall peaked P waves are an indication of right atrial enlargement, which is typically caused by high right atrial pressures. Increased CO wouldn't cause RAE, and neither would reduced SVR, reduced CVP, nor hyperkalemia. If you choose hyperkalemia, remember that hyperkalemia causes a peaked T waves, not peaked P waves.

6. (**B**) Understanding the components of the cardiac cycle is imperative for these certification exams. When the AV valve closes, it makes a dull 'thump' sound that we recognize as the "lub" sound, also known as the S1 heart tone. Lub-Dub is equivalent to the S1 and S2 respectively.

7. (**B**) A Q wave that is either greater than 1/3 the height of the R wave or > 0.03 of a second (or 30 milliseconds) is indicative of a pathological q wave, therefore, this is the correct answer.

8. (**C**) To answer this question, you'll need to know how to identify left and right bundle branches. Left bundle branch blocks can be identified by a wide QRS complex (> 120ms) and a downward deflection from the J point (retrograde in direction) on a 12 lead ECG. Right bundle branch blocks can be identified by a wide QRS complex (> 120ms) and an upward deflection from the J point (retrograde in direction) on a 12 lead ECG.

9. (**D**) Three criteria are included in Sgarbossa's criteria: (1) ST elevation ≥1 mm in a lead with a positive QRS complex [i.e.: concordance] earns 5 points; (2) ST depression ≥1 mm in lead V1, V2, or V3 earns 3 points; (3) ST elevation ≥5 mm in a lead with a negative [discordant] QRS complex earns 2 points. When ≥3 points are earned, there is a 90% specificity of STEMI (sensitivity of 36%). So, in this case there is 8 points earned, confirming a current STEMI from concordance in V6 (upright QRS with ST elevation earning 5 points) and concordance in V3 (negative QRS and ST depression earning 3 points).

10. (**B**) To identify a biatrial enlargement, you need to identify a biphasic p wave in V1 as well as either p- mitrale (M- shaped p wave) or p- pulmonale (tall peaked p wave). This needs to be committed to memory.

11. (**A**) It indicates left ventricular hypertrophy. For LVH to be present, there are multiple criteria. This question presents answers referring to the Deep/ tall criteria. If the deepest S wave (V1 or V2) plus the tallest R wave (in V5 or V6) is 35 mm or higher, then LVH is present. In this question only one answer matches this this criteria is the answer: V2 S wave and V6 R wave together is 37 mm. Remember, it's S depth in V1 or V2 PLUS the R height in V5 or V6; if it's > 35 mm high then LVH is present.

12. (**A**) This is a simple recall question. You need to recognize that preload, afterload, and contractility are VERY much related, and specifically relate to stroke volume (or the amount of blood ejected by the heart per beat). Decreasing preload and contractility will both DECREASE stroke volume. Increasing afterload will DECREASE stroke volume. Conversely, increasing preload and contractility will INCREASE stroke volume and, as expected, reducing afterload will INCREASE stroke volume.

13. (**A**) This is another important question to be able to answer. You'll need to know the coronary artery reach and which coronary artery goes with what area on the 12 ECG. This area is fed by the left anterior coronary artery- here mentioned as the left coronary artery.

14. (**C**) Look at the CVP pressures, or otherwise recognize the CVP waveform- it goes from low to MUCH higher. This occurs when the PA catheter that is sitting in the right atrium accidentally migrates into the right ventricle. The right ventricle HATEs this and can start through PVCs or runs of VTACH. Therefore, this is the PA cath migrating from the right atrium (RA) to the right

ventricle (RV). To correct this, deflate and withdraw the balloon out of the right ventricle.

15. (**D**) Dilated cardiomyopathy patients are treated just like heart failure patients: heart failure management with CPAP, nitrates, loop diuretics, morphine, ACE inhibitors, inotropes.

16. (**A**) The typical ST elevation MI (or STEMI) involves ST elevation changes. These changes occur in a pattern as the MI runs its course. They progress through (1) hyperacute T wave phase, (2) acute phase 1, (3) acute phase 2, and (4) age indeterminate phase. The key feature in hyperacute T waves is: hyperacute T waves (shocker). With possible ST depression. In the acute phase I progression phase, the key feature is an elevated ST segment. The key feature in the acute phase II progression phase is the introduction of pathological Q waves and residual ST segment elevation (residual ST segment elevation from acute phase I). The Age Indeterminate phase of MI progression, the key feature is a pathological Q wave WITHOUT any ST elevation. Therefore the correct answer selection for this question is acute phase I- because there is ST elevation in the absence of a pathological Q wave.

17. (**A**) In this patient, there is a high CVP, which directly indicates a WET SYSTEM. Heart failure (right side issues in this case) prevent easy, forward flow, thus a back pressure occurs backwards from the right side of the heart. The left heart is not affected (normal PCWP), therefore, the lungs are dry in this case. Recap: High CVP means wet system and a high PCWP means wet lungs.

18. (**D**) The ECG ST elevation pattern (V5, V6, aVL and lead I) in this question is specific to an lateral/ high lateral wall AMI. These AMIs occur mostly from a blockage of the left anterior descending artery and left circumflex (MOSTLY) arteries.

19. (**C**) Before you treat an aortic dissection with vasodilators, you need to treat with a medication that reduces the force of the velocity of the blood being ejected out of the heart. High ejection pressures further tear the dissection. Therefore, slow down that velocity with a negative inotrope (like a beta blocker- which is common) before adding a vasodilator.

20. (**B**) Levophed is a medication that is a catecholamine, or a chemical that mimics epinephrine to varying degrees. Levophed highly stimulates alpha 1 and slightly stimulates beta 1, therefore, BP will go up primarily (from increased SVR) and with it the HR will increase (which increases CO and BP a little). Here, the "Increased HR and blood pressure" is the correct answer.

21. (**B**) If the patient has a dual pacer, then where is the pacer spikes on the ventricular beat? In this case, there is no ventricular pacer spike, so we have failure to capture. We don't have the information to identify if hypoxia is occurring, nor do we have enough information to identify if a left bundle branch block is present. Finally, these are pacer spikes, not pointed p-waves.

22. (**D**) A CO of 6 L/min is normal and indicates that the IABP has been successful in treating the shock.

23. (**C**) It is important to know ALL of the value ranges for the various cardiac parameters. In this case, you are asked to know the ranges for core body temperature (which is 98.6 degrees, or about 37 degrees Celsius), cardiac output (which is 4-8 L/min), and blood pressure (which is typically perfusing when above 90 systolic). The only one that seems dangerous is the low cardiac output, because 3 L/min for an adult is way too low- that patient is dry as hell. Fluid, fluid, fluid. The temperature is 0.6 degrees F low, but that isn't enough to call it 'dangerous'.

24. (**A**) There is only one medication in the answer selections that act as a vasodilator, and that's nitroglycerine. Please note that the CVP and PCWP are both high- meaning there is fluid backing up on both sides of the heart and thus requiring a relief of this pressure. To relieve this pressure and correct the hemodynamics in this situation, nitro can be administered to act as a vasodilator. This would reduce afterload by making the arteries larger and thus will help relieve the increased intracardiac pressure.

25. (**D**) It is important to know ALL of the value ranges for the various cardiac parameters. In this case, you need to know not only the normal range of cardiac output, but you need to know the cardiac output for each of the major age ranges: adult, pediatric, and infant. Adult is 4-8 L/min, pediatric is 1-3 L/min, and an infant is 0.8-1 L/min. The only patient in the question that is exhibiting abnormal hemodynamics is the 22 y/o trauma patient. Trauma patients' mortality drastically increase with a single episode of hypotension- this 22 y/o has a low cardiac output, suggesting he needs lots of fluids.

26. (**D**) Notching with ST elevation is most likely 100% NOT an acute MI, therefore, the 'AMI is absent' answer selection is the correct answer.

27. (**D**) To answer this question you need to understand what information the question is offering you. SUDDEN onset of shortness of breath should put PE on your radar. The S/ R wave data should prompt you to investigate for LVH or RVH. Any time R and S wave heights are provided, apply your hypertrophy criterias to identify if hypertrophy is present. Then recall what are common causes of these hypertrophies. In this case, RVH is present (because in V1 the R wave is bigger than the S wave). RVH is caused by anything that prevents blood flow through the lungs- resulting in back pressure (like a PE). Contused lungs would swell and reduce blood flow through

them, thus increasing the pressures in the right side of the heart, and boom- RVH. Congestive HF is close, but the onset probably wouldn't be sudden-it would probably be gradual. Asthmaticus is more an airway issue, instead of vascular.

28. (**B**) Look at the very noticeable dicrotic notch following the systolic peak. The dicrotic notch begins, ends, and then the balloon is inflated. The dicrotic notch is COMPLETELY visible. This is clear late inflation.

29. (**C**) High CO and low SVR with mostly normal other hemodynamic parameters, is difficult to diagnose confidently. However, if there is evidence of fever/ shock, then the diagnosis becomes clear. Here, the patient returns 3 days after surgery diaphoretic (probably because they are warm/hot with fever), which suggests sepsis by itself, but add it to the high cardiac output with a low SVR, it's a dead giveaway for septic shock. Remember, high temp and CO with low SVR is strongly suggestive of septic shock. This is a type of distributive shock, but the more specific choice is septic shock, therefore distributive is not the MOST correct answer.

30. (**B**) The inferior wall is mostly fed by the right coronary artery. Memorize these.

31. (**A**) Administration of Levophed stimulates both the alpha 1 and beta 1 receptors. By stimulating the alpha 1 receptor, you will increase vasoconstriction (with raises blood pressure). By stimulating the beta 1 receptor you increase HR via increasing SA node firing (chronotropy) and increasing the speed through which electrical impulses travel through the conductive system (dromotropy). Additionally, beta 1 stimulation increases cardiac contractility, but that isn't a factor in this question since there isn't any mention of contractility in the answer selections.

32. (**B**) To answer this question, you'll need to know the

morphology of digitalis toxicity. It presents with a "ladle effect" which looks like a concave ST segment to the right of the QRS complex. This is specific to digitalis toxicity.

33. (**D**) Neosynepherine is almost all alpha 1. This medication will increase blood pressure by causing vasoconstriction, therefore the measured SVR will increase. Neosynepherine will not directly increase CVP, nor will it reduce PVR or cardiac output.

34. (**D**) To answer this question you'll have to be able to identify the criteria of a bundle branch block. The main criteria taught in my text is a prolonged QRS waveform. Prolonged QRS is defined as greater than 120ms, or longer than 3 small ECG boxes. In this case, the answer of 4 small QRS boxes is correct because that means that the impulse takes 160ms to get through the conductive tissue (40ms per small box). It is important to be able to describe the same concept in different ways, such as here where 120ms actually equals 3 small boxes.

35. (**B**) Here the only value that is not within its normal limits is the BICARBONATE of 31. Bicarbonate should be in the ball park of 22-26 [mEq/L]. All the other values are within normal limits.

36. (**C**) You will need to be able to identify pericarditis to be able to answer this question. Pericarditis presents with global ST elevation, PR depression (exhibited here as PR segment below the isoelectric line), notching of the QRS, and a scooping and upward concave ST segment. Additionally, if you see ST elevation in Lead I and II, then be suspicious for pericarditis.

37. (**A**) To answer this question you need to understand how cardiac output is affected by heart rate and by stroke volume. CO= HR x SV, so any increase in HR or stroke volume will INCREASE cardiac output. Therefore, and decrease in HR or SV will DECREASE cardiac output. We know that bradycardia is a HR less than 60, therefore the patient most likely experienced a

drop in cardiac output.

38. (**B**) This is a characteristic finding in the **LATE DEFLATION**. Refer to Section 1, Chapter 6, Part 9 in Swearingen's Resource and Study Guide for Critical Care Transport Clinicians.

39. (**B**) In treating AMI, or any active MI for that matter, ASA will prevent further sticking of platelets, nitro will act as a vasodilator (especially on the coronary arteries), heparin thins out the blood so the heart doesn't have to pump as hard to propel the blood forward, and beta blockers slower the hearts efforts to reduce myocardial oxygen demand. This patient most likely could benefit from some fluid, as long as there wasn't rales or crackles- which ever the term of the month for "wet lungs" is. Warfarin and Versed aren't indicated.

40. (**D**) This question is illustrating an age indeterminate phase of an AMI. Pathological Q waves indicate a previous AMI (meaning the patient is predisposed to it). In the acute phase I progression phase, the key feature is an elevated ST segment. The key feature in hyperacute T waves is: hyperacute T waves (shocker). With possible ST depression. The key feature in the acute phase II progression phase is the introduction of pathological Q waves and residual ST segment elevation (residual ST segment elevation from acute phase I). The Age Indeterminate phase of MI progression, the key feature is a pathological Q wave WITHOUT any ST elevation. Therefore the correct answer selection for this question is age indeterminate- since there is only a pathologic Q waves observed in the presence of chest pain and elevated cardiac enzymes.

41. (**A**) The lateral wall is fed mostly by the left circumflex (MOSTLY) and the left anterior descending. Memorize these.

42. (**A**) The condition described is pulmonary edema, which is found MOST SPECIFICALLY with left sided heart failure. Congestive

heart failure might be a tempting answer selection, but it is not the best answer in this case because congestive heart failure consists of BOTH left and right heart failure findings (thus congestive = both sides in failure). In this case, the right sided symptoms are absent (JVD and acietes).

43. (**B**) Cardiac Output = HR x SV. So, if you know both HR and CO, then you can calculate the SV. This has been asked on critical care certification exams, even though it really doesn't change our care. I included it to make sure you have seen it. In this case, SV = (CO/HR), or SV = 5400/105 = 51 mL.

44. (**A**) Normally, CVP is 2-8 mmHg, SVR is 800-1300 dynes/sec/cm^3, PCWP is 4-12 mmHg, and CO is normally 4-8 L/min. Therefore, the only one in its normal range in this case is the PCWP of 11.

45. (**D**) The Sgarbossa criteria is a method of assessing chest pain patients with left bundle branch blocks (LBBBs) for an active AMI.

46. (**C**) Here the only value that is not within its normal limits is the HEMATOCRIT of 29. The hematocrit should be about 45% (39-49% for males and 35-45% for females]. WBC is about 4.5-11, HBG 12-17.5, HCT 34-52, and platelets 150-450. These are rough guidelines, so please be sure to memorize your specific institution where you work.

47. (**C**) Hypovolemic shock presents with low CVP and PCWP, normal or low CO, but for sure presents with high SVR- so most everything is low, or low side of normal, but SVR is high. Here CVP, PCWP are both low with the CO on the low side of normal, while the SVR is extremely high, thus represents HYPOVOLEMIC shock.

48. (**C**) PCWP (or wedge pressure) effects left ventricular end diastolic pressure (or left ventricular preload). Because the patient in left ventricular failure will have a high PCWP (as is the

case with the option "wedge pressure of 16"), a decrease in this value will be the best indicator of patient improvement. The other values would also provide useful information, but the most definitive measurement of improvement is a drop in PCWP.

49. (**B**) Understanding the components of the cardiac cycle is imperative for these certification exams. When the AV valve closes, it makes a dull 'thump' sound that we recognize as the "lub" sound, also known as the S1 heart tone. When the semilunar valves close (the pulmonic and aortic valves), then the "dub' sound is generated. Lub-Dub is equivalent to the S1 and S2 respectively. S3 and S4 are extra sounds caused by various conditions. S3 occurs with S1 and S2, but the way that it is generated it presents with an S1, followed by S2 and S3 that are very close together. This makes the KEN----tuck-y sound that is mentioned in this literature. This indicates heart failure or volume overload. The S4 sound is heard BEFORE S1 and progresses as follows: S4 and S1 very close together, a short pause, and then the S2 sound. This gives the characteristic pattern similar to saying the word: TEN-NES----ee. This occurs from forcing blood into a failing or hypertrophic left heart.

50. (**C**) The ECG ST elevation pattern (elevation in V1 and V2) in this question is specific to an septal wall AMI. These AMIs occur mostly from a blockage of the left anterior descending artery.

51. (**B**) WPW presents with a delta wave, which is identified by a shortened PR segment (from a reentry pathway) which then creates a delta shape and a lengthy QRS. The two factors that identifies the delta wave is the short PR segment (< 120 milliseconds) and a long QRS (or at least not a short one) at < 100 milliseconds.

52. (**C**) High and peaked T waves occur clinically with a K+ of typically 5.5 or above. Digitalis toxicity presents with the ladle

effect morphology and normal levels are usually 0.6-.08 ng/dL. Hypercalcemia essentially has rounded T-wave 12 lead morphology. The correct answer is a potassium of 6.1.

53. (**B**) Look at the very noticeable dicrotic notch following the systolic peak. The dicrotic notch begins, ends, and then the balloon is inflated. The dicrotic notch is COMPLETELY visible. This is clear late inflation.

54. (**A**) The two most common etiologies of cardiac tamponade is pericarditis and chest trauma. Therefore, if you come across a pericarditis patient, routinely rule out signs/ symptoms of tamponade. If you are looking for this stuff, you'll catch things earlier.

55. (**B**) The BP is out of normal limits, but is not an answer selection. The only other number out of range, and thus concerning, is the SVR. Normal SVR is 800- 1200 dynes/sec/cm^3. At 1500, there is some serious AFTERLOAD happening (very high). This means the heart has to work extra hard to push blood out of the left ventricle against the high pressures (from afterload).

56. (**B**) This patient has a left axis deviation (upright waveform in lead I and a negative waveform in aVF). A left axis deviation also means there is a conduction block of the left anterior hemifasicle, or also known as hemiblock. To be able to answer this question, you'll have to be able to know the criteria for axis deviation. Normal is lead I and aVF are positive. Left axis deviation is where lead I is positive and aVF is negative. Right axis is where lead I is negative and aVF is positive. Extreme axis deviation is where both lead I and aVF are both negative.

57. (**D**) The ECG ST elevation pattern (elevation in V3 and V4 with possible ST depression in V8 and V9) in this question is specific to an anterior wall AMI. These AMIs occur mostly from a blockage of the left anterior descending artery.

58. (**C**) For LVH to be present, there are multiple criteria. This question presents answers referring to the aVL criteria. Under this criteria, if the aVL R wave is larger than 11mm then LVH is present. In this question the correct answer is the only one meeting this criteria: aVL R wave is 12 mm.

59. (**D**) In cardiogenic shock, some pathophysiology damages the heart, or prevents it from functioning normally. This weakens the pump. With a weak pump the heart cannot produce enough pressure to perfuse the distal tissues (skin, brain, liver, lungs, etc). This poor perfusion leads to widespread acidosis and, if uncorrected, death.

60. (**D**) This is an APPROPRIATE positioning. The AP chest should the IABP balloon at about the 2nd or 3rd intercostal space, which places it 1-2 cm under the subclavian artery and also above the renal arteries. If placed to low (like at the 5th intercostal space) then it occludes the renal arteries, and if placed too high it will occlude the subclavian, brachiocephalic, and carotid arteries.

61. (**C**) This is early deflation. This doesn't directly hurt the patient, but also doesn't exactly help. It results in reduced inflation time leading to lower peak diastolic augmentation time and sub-optimal IABP functioning. This also could potentially cause a retrograde coronary blood flow leading to angina, arrhythmias, and potentially AMI.

62. (**B**) The ECG ST elevation pattern (elevation in II, III, and aVF with possible ST depression in I and aVL) in this question is specific to an inferior wall AMI. These AMIs occur mostly from a blockage of the right coronary artery.

63. (**A**) A low CVP (less than 2 mmHg as is in this case) indicates hypovolemia and a need for an increase in the infusion rate. Diuretic administration will contribute to hypovolemia and

elevation of the head may decrease cerebral perfusion. Documentation and continued monitoring is an inadequate response to the low CVP. The goal is to increase the CVP to normal levels and to ensure an adequate urinary output (~ 0.5 - 1.0 cc/kg/hr).

64. (**B**) All the hemodynamic parameters are high except one: cardiac output. This is very tell- tale for cardiogenic shock. It makes sense too, right? The heart is busted, so it cannot push blood forward. This causes a backup which leads to building pressure. High pressures and not a lot being pushed forward = cardiogenic shock.

65. (**C**) Dopamine administered in the middle dosing range (5-10 mcg/kg/min will elicit a mixed adrenergic effect (meaning it will stimulate more than one receptor). At this dose it will stimulate both alpha 1 and beta 1. This results in an increased CO and increased BP (from ↑ SVR). With the answer choices available, the best answer is ↑ SVR. At this dose a little ↑ pulmonary vascular resistance PVR) can occur and perhaps a little indirect ↑ PCWP, but the most direct actions are from ↑ SVR.

66. (**C**) This patient is suffering from neurogenic shock (fractured neck with a demarcation line on the skin illustrating massive vasodilation). Fluids are needed, but a pressor is also needed to take control of the vasoconstriction because the cut nerves below the injury no longer can stimulate vasoconstriction- thus we have to give medicine to make vasoconstriction occur. If you only administer fluids, then the patient most likely would remain hypotension due to lack of neurologic control of the peripheral blood vessels. Here the SVR is extremely low- we can fix it with a pressor.

67. (**B**) Normally, systolic RVP is 25-30 mmHg, diastolic RVP is 0-5 mmHg, systolic PAP is 15-30 mmHg, and diastolic PAP is 5-10 mmHg, therefore, the only answer selection here that is within

normal limits is the diastolic PAP of 9.

68. (**D**) The condition is cardiac tamponade: fluid accumulating between the pericardium and the pericardial sac.

69. (**B**) This question is testing your knowledge on axis deviation. You'll need to know how to identify axis deviation. Normal is lead I and aVF are positive. Left axis deviation is where lead I is positive and aVF is negative. Right axis is where lead I is negative and aVF is positive. Extreme axis deviation is where both lead I and aVF are both negative.

70. (**D**) Normally, systolic RVP is 25-30 mmHg, diastolic RVP is 0-5 mmHg, systolic PAP is 15-30 mmHg, and diastolic PAP is 5-10 mmHg, therefore, the only answer selection here that is within normal limits is the systolic RVP of 30.

71. (**D**) An M- shaped p wave indicates left atrial enlargement. This is commonly caused by a diseased mitral valve. Therefore, answer choices right atrial enlargement and diseased tricuspid valve is incorrect. This also doesn't meet the criteria for a silent AMI. P mitrale is also known as left atrial enlargement- therefore this is the correct answer.

72. (**C**) There are 2 types of VADs with regard to flow- pulsatile (produces pulse) and continuous flow (doesn't create a pulse). The best approach with VAD and cardiovascular pathophysiologies is to allow their mental status and perfusion status guide your concerns. If the patient is calm and following commands without a pulse or in v-tach, then just apply supportive treatment as opposed to drastic ACLS protocols.

73. (**A**) In this case, supportive care (fluid bolus and monitoring) is all that is warranted. Remember, this patient has his blood being pumped by the machine essentially, so protect with supportive care (oxygen/ fluid) as long as their mental state and perfusion state are adequate- ensured here by a and awake

patient with good capillary refill.

74. (**C**) Notice the pattern of ST elevation in leads II, III, and aVF. This is typical of inferior wall AMI.

75. (**C**) Notice the pattern of ST elevation in leadsV1 –V4. This is typical of antrioseptal wall AMI.

76. (**D**) Notice the pattern of ST depression in V2 and V3 with tall R waves. This suggests <u>posterior wall AMI</u>. A right sided MI and V4R, V5R, and V6R should be run.

7 RESPIRATORY

Questions

1. As you are packaging our patient, the RN returns with the following ABG: pH 7.46/ pCO2 44/ HCO3 43/ pO2 87/ BE 2. Interpret these findings.

   A. Metabolic alkalosis
   B. Respiratory alkalosis
   C. Metabolic acidosis
   D. Respiratory acidosis

2. Your patient presents with difficulty breathing, anxiety, and wheezing, RR 28 and shallow, no breath sounds, and a diminishing mental status. She has been treated with continuous B2 agonists and anticholinergics. Which of the following would be the next most appropriate treatment?

   A. Admin racemic epinephrine
   B. Apply BiPAP without PEEP
   C. Intubate with only paralytics
   D. 2g of Mag over 20 minutes

3. An ARDS patient is to be transferred to a larger tertiary hospital. Which of the following common therapies are successful in the management of ARDS?

   A. Administer high tidal volumes to patient
   B. Deliver high FiO2; maintain low EtCO2
   C. Reverse I:E; permissive hypercapnia
   D. Ensure the pO2 is at about 50 mmHg

4. You are noticing a change in the patients' status. Upon and arterial blood draw and analysis, you obtain the following ABG: pH 7.21/ pCO2 61/ HCO3 22/ pO2 120/ BE 0. What degree of compensation is present here, if any?

   A. This is a MIXED problem
   B. This is an ACUTE problem
   C. Partially compensated
   D. Fully compensated

5. After establishing your initial vent settings and one vent change, you notice the SpO2 is 88%. Which of the following is the best management for this patient?

   A. Increase PEEP
   B. Increase rate
   C. Increase the TV
   D. Increase the PC

6. You are treating a patient with severe shortness of breath with wheezing. Currently their oxygen saturation is 88% and they have the following arterial blood gas data: 7.31/ CO2 56/ HCO3 23. What is the next most appropriate action to perform on this patient?

   A. Intubation
   B. Magnesium
   C. Terbutaline
   D. Epinephrine

7. Your patient has the following vital signs: BP 134/88, HR 92, EtCO2 61, SpO2 94%. Which of the following would cause these vital signs?

   A. Hypothermia
   B. Dislodged ETT
   C. Bicarb admin
   D. Pulm. Embolus

8. You are examining a patient before you begin the packaging process, and notice that their EtCO2 is 49 mmHg. How would you best correct this problem?

   A. Change FiO2 from 1 to 0.7
   B. Change TV from 600 to 450
   C. Change PEEP from 5 to 3
   D. Change RR from 12 to 16

9. You notice your patient has an increasing EtCO2. The astute critical care clinician knows to asses which of the following?

   A. CNS depression
   B. Ca administration
   C. ↑ minute volume
   D. Pre-cardiac arrest

10. Look at the provided chest x-rays. What are the arrows pointing to?

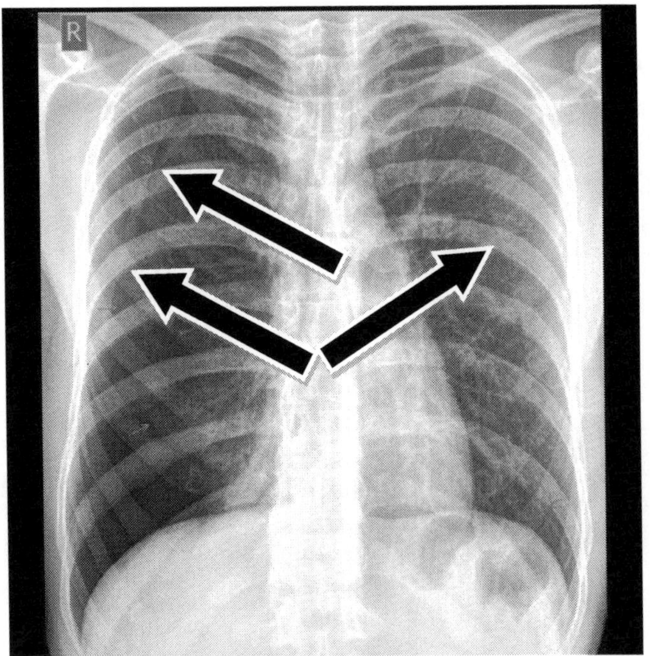

   A. A collapsed lung
   B. Wide mediastinum
   C. Cardiac tamponade
   D. Cardiomegaly

11. A chronically ill patient has the following ABG: pH 7.29/ pCO_2 49/ HCO_3 30/ pO_2 98/ BE 1. What degree of compensation is present here, if any?

    A. This is a MIXED problem
    B. Fully compensated
    C. This is an ACUTE problem
    D. Partially compensated

12. Your COPD patient presents with difficult breathing. The physician has requested you perform a trial of non-invasive positive pressure ventilation. Which of the following are the most appropriate initial settings?

    A. PS of 12, PEEP 5
    B. IPAP 10, EPAP 0
    C. IPAP 25, EPAP 0
    D. PS of 5, PEEP 5

13. Originally, the ABG on your respiratory distress patient was as follows: 7.32/ CO_2 49/ HCO_3 22. At this time the potassium was 4.5 mmHg. The new ABG is as follows: 7.22/ CO_2 59/ HCO_3 21. Which of the following potassium values would be correct following this change?

    A. 5.1 mmol/L
    B. 3.9 mmol/L
    C. 4.8 mEq/L
    D. 4.2 mEq/L

14. You are transporting a trauma patient to a trauma center. Earlier, they has oxygen saturations of100% on room air, but now their oxygen saturation is 90%. What would you expect their PaO2 at this time?

    A. 80 mmHg
    B. 70 mmHg
    C. 60 mmHg
    D. 50 mmHg

15. An asthma patient is on the mechanical ventilator. You hear a ventilator alarm and observe the following: volume control, SIMV, RR 18, Vt 450, I:E 1:2, PEEP 5, FiO2 1.0, f 18, Vte 300, PIP 65, Pplat 22, AutoPEEP 3, EtCO2 is 54. Which of the following is the most appropriate approach?

    A. Increase the RR
    B. Extend the E time
    C. Extend the I time
    D. Increase the Vt

16. As you are looking over your intubated patient's chart, you notice the following ABG: pH 7.32/ pCO2 46/ HCO3 20/ pO2 87/ BE 0. What degree of compensation is present here, if any?

    A. Partially compensated
    B. This is an ACUTE problem
    C. This is a MIXED problem
    D. Fully compensated

17. The patient you are transporting to the regional hospital presents with the following ABG: pH 7.47/ pCO2 25/ HCO3 25/ pO2 89/ BE 1. Interpret these findings.

A. Respiratory acidosis
B. Metabolic alkalosis
C. Metabolic acidosis
D. Respiratory alkalosis

18. Your transporting a motor vehicle collision patient from the scene to a level one trauma center. The accident happened approximately 1 hour ago and the patient was just extricated 10 minutes ago. The ambient temperature is near freezing. Which of the following findings would you most likely see with this patient?

A. Profound hypotension from the ambient temp
B. Slurring of the QRS evident on the 12 lead ECG
C. Left shift of oxyhemoglobin disassociation curve
D. Significant DIC from being entrapped for 50 min

19. Your intubated patient is on a mechanical ventilator, and you notice the following findings: HR 101, SpO2 94%,MV 3.5 L/min, EtCO2 55, and a Vte of 450 cc. What do these values tell you about the oxyhemoglobin disassociation curve?

A. There is a shift to the left
B. There is a shift to the right
C. Reduction in oxygen supply
D. Reduction in oxygen demand

20. A patient with acute respiratory distress syndrome is being transported to an ICU. You have them on the mechanical ventilator as follows: PC 20, PEEP of 20, RR 14, FiO2 of 1.0 on assist control. The patient's SpO2 is still incredibly low. Which of the following could improve the patient's oxygen saturations?

A. Reduce PEEP
B. Increase MV
C. Raise the TV
D. Reverse I:E

21. On your way to an Interfacility transfer, you receive word that your respiratory failure patient has the following ABG: pH 7.22/ pCO2 47/ HCO3 29/ pO2 82/ BE 0. Interpret these findings.

A. Respiratory acidosis
B. Metabolic acidosis
C. Respiratory alkalosis
D. Metabolic alkalosis

22. You are dispatched to a local hospital where your patient has the following ABG: pH 7.33/ pCO2 45/ HCO3 20/ pO2 83/ BE 1. Interpret these findings.

A. Respiratory acidosis
B. Metabolic acidosis
C. Respiratory alkalosis
D. Metabolic alkalosis

23. You are orienting a new employee and mention an ABG that you recently had on a flight: pH 7.35/ pCO2 50/ HCO3 29/ pO2 87/ BE 1. What degree of compensation is present here, if any?

A. This is an ACUTE problem
B. Partially compensated
C. Fully compensated
D. This is a MIXED problem

24. A patient has been intubated for an altered mental status. He has the following clinical findings: SIMV, RR 12, VT 390, FIO2 100% PEEP 4, Vte 375, and (f) 28. The vital signs are BP 122/672, HR 64, SPO2 96%, and EtC02 28. Which of the following is the most appropriate action?

A. Increase the patient's Vt
B. Change the patient's RR
C. Administer sedative
D. Manually bag patient

25. Your medical patient is currently receiving mechanical ventilation with a current PEEP setting of 5 cmH2O. Which of the following statements is TRUE regarding PEEP?

A. It is mostly applied during inspiration
B. It thins the alveolar capillary membrane
C. It increases inspiratory reserve capacity
D. It causes cardiac output to elevate

26. Your vent patient has the following clinical findings: SIMV 15 (f 21), VT 425, FIO2 100% PEEP 4. The vital signs are BP 136/88, HR 99, SPO2 98%, and EtC02 32. Which of the following is the most appropriate action?

A. Increate the RR
B. Reduce the FiO2
C. Manually bag patient
D. Administer versed

27. You are explaining the mechanical ventilator to a new hire. You explain how to apply the SIMV mode. You know that this mode will do which of the following?

A. Allow the patient to breathe on their own
B. Synchronize with each exhaled breath
C. Requires a paralytic be administered early
D. Causes PEEP to rise with each breath

28. Your adult trauma patient is intubated and has the following ventilator settings: A/C, RR 11, VT 460, FIO2 100%, PEEP 4. His vital signs are BP 124/76, HR 70, SPO2 98%, ETCO2 52. The next most appropriate action is to?

A. Raise the RR to 14
B. Adjust the Vt to 425
C. Adjust the PEEP to 6
D. Reduce FiO2 to 0.7

29. While caring for a patient who is mechanically ventilated and on positive end-expiratory pressure (PEEP), it is important to understand how PEEP works. Which of the following statements is TRUE regarding PEEP?

A. It occurs at the beginning of a machine breath
B. It decreases the functional residual capacity (FRC)
C. It causes an increased venous return
D. It may reduce minute ventilation (VE)

30. Your partner tells you they have set up the ventilator on pressure control ventilation at 17/5 on 100% oxygen with normal I:E. This information tells you what about your patient?

A. Their peak pressure is now 12
B. The pressure control is 22
C. The minute ventilation is 6L/min
D. The I:E is appropriate for the pt

31. While caring for a patient who is mechanically ventilated and on positive end-expiratory pressure (PEEP). Which of the following statements is TRUE regarding PEEP?

A. It is applied during spontaneous inspiration involving SIMV

B. It increases the surface area of the alveolar membrane

C. It dramatically increases the patient's inspiratory reserve

D. It causes an increased venous return and cardiac output

Answers

1. (**A**) Step 1- last name- is pH acidotic or alkalotic? Step 2- middle name- which sub-parameter matches the pH.- if PaCO2 matches then its "respiratory" as middle name and if HCO3 matches then the middle name is "metabolic". Step 3- ID level of compensation- acute (if pH and one sub-parameter match and the other sub-parameter is NORMAL), Mixed (all parameters either acidic or alkalotic), Partially compensated (if 3 No Rule present), and Fully compensation (if pH is normal and both sub-parameters are abnormal).

2. (**D**) This patient needs to be intubated and magnesium is indicated (since this is a severe asthma exacerbation). You shouldn't intubate awake people with ONLY a paralytic, so that answer selection is wrong. BiPAP without PEEP is impossible since the lower pressure (CPAP) is also PEEP. Yes, CPAP and PEEP are EXACTLY the same thing. Racemic epinephrine is not indicated here.

3. (**C**) Common practices to minimize overdistention and damage to lung tissue for patients in ARDS, is to reverse the I:E ratio (example: 2:1). This increases E time and therefore drops the PIP. Longer I times means the air has a longer, slower time to inhale resulting in lower PIPs. Placing the patient in PC ventilation also controls for lower PIPs as well, but wasn't an answer here. Avoid delivering very high FiO2 because it can further damage

tissues. High tidal volumes can injure the patient.

4. (**B**) Step 1- last name- is pH acidotic or alkalotic? Step 2- middle name- which sub-parameter matches the pH.- if $PaCO_2$ matches then its "respiratory" as middle name and if HCO_3 matches then the middle name is "metabolic". Step 3- ID level of compensation- acute (if pH and one sub-parameter match and the other sub-parameter is NORMAL), Mixed (all parameters either acidic or alkalotic), Partially compensated (if 3 No Rule present), and Fully compensation (if pH is normal and both sub-parameters are abnormal).

5. (**A**) The only settings that can effectively effect a change in SpO_2 is increasing or decreasing PEEP and/ or FiO_2. While I time will also increase oxygenation, in transport this text will argue that the best way to improve SpO_2 is to increase PEEP or FiO_2.

6. (**A**) Once the CO_2 gets above 55 mmHg, then intubation is indicated in shortness of breath patients that are refractory to other treatments. The other medications are all appropriate but at this point the patient needs to be intubated.

7. (**C**) Once bicarb is administered (typically during severe acidosis) excess CO_2 is formed almost instantly, resulting in an immediate increase in end-tidal carbon dioxide tension. Hypothermia, dislodged endotracheal tube (ETT), and PEs all will reduce the measured $EtCO_2$.

8. (**D**) The only settings that can change $EtCO_2$ is TV, RR, and pressure control. Increasing TV, RR, and PC will REDUCE $EtCO_2$ while decreasing TV, RR, and PC will all

ELEVATE EtCO2. Changing the RR from 12 to 16 would help reduce the EtCO2, therefore it is the correct answer.

9. (**A**) Central nervous system (CNS) depression will result in reduced minute volume from a reduced RR. This will cause a rise in EtCO2. Calcium administration will not cause a direct rise in EtCO2. Increased minute volume (aka minute ventilation) and pre-cardiac arrest states will reduce cardiac output as well as EtCO2.

10. (**A**) The arrows are pointing to collapsed lungs, or pneumothoracies.

11. (**D**) Step 1- last name- is pH acidotic or alkalotic? Step 2- middle name- which sub-parameter matches the pH.- if PaCO2 matches then its "respiratory" as middle name and if HCO3 matches then the middle name is "metabolic". Step 3- ID level of compensation- acute (if pH and one sub-parameter match and the other sub-parameter is NORMAL), Mixed (all parameters either acidic or alkalotic), Partially compensated (if 3 No Rule present), and Fully compensation (if pH is normal and both sub-parameters are abnormal).

12. (**A**) PS and IPAP are the same thing with an additive bi-level positive airway pressure ventilator. The literature suggest 8-12 cmH2O of PS and suggests an EPAP, or PEEP, of 4-5 cmH2O. This makes the "PS of 12, PEEP 5" answer selection correct. EPAP shouldn't start at zero and you wouldn't set an IPAP without an EPAP and two answers have a zero for EPAP. Remember, the IPAP is the PS + PEEP, or said another way, the PS + EPAP.

13. (**A**) Every change in pH of 0.1, the potassium changes 0.6 in the opposite direction. Therefore if pH is 7.32 and changes to 7.22 (a reduction), then the potassium will increase. If it started out at 4.5 mmol/L, then it would be 5.1 mmol/L after the change in pH.

14. (**C**) If the monitored SpO2 is 90%, then the expected PaCO2 is 60 mmHg. If the monitored SpO2 is 80%, then the expected PaCO2 is 50 mmHg. If the monitored SpO2 is 70%, then the expected PaCO2 is 40 mmHg. Commit these to memory.

15. (**B**) The most appropriate thing to do here would be to reduce the rate, but its not an option. The patient has a positive AutoPEEP (meaning they are air trapping). AutoPEEP should be zero, and a positive number indicates air trapping. Air trapping can cause the Vte to be lower than the set tidal volume (due to trapped air). To prevent this, you need to either increase the exhalation time (to allow the trapped gas to escape) or you need to reduce the RR (which happens to also lengthen the E time and thus exhalation time). Increasing the I time will SHORTEN the E time, so that's a wrong answer. Increasing either RR or Vt will drop the EtCO2, but first always **clear out the trapped gas** by lowering RR or increasing the E time. If you do not clear out trapped gas and instead increase the RR or Vt (tidal volume) then you will be prolonging dangerous alveolar distention and worsening hypercapnia.

16. (**C**) This is a MIXED problem because thr pH, pCO2, and HCO3 all are acidic like. Step 1- last name- is pH acidotic or alkalotic? Step 2- middle name- which sub-parameter

matches the pH.- if PaCO2 matches then its "respiratory" as middle name and if HCO3 matches then the middle name is "metabolic". Step 3- ID level of compensation- acute (if pH and one sub-parameter match and the other sub-parameter is NORMAL), Mixed (all parameters either acidic or alkalotic), Partially compensated (if 3 No Rule present), and Fully compensation (if pH is normal and both sub-parameters are abnormal).

17. (**D**) Respiratory alkalosis. Step 1- last name- is pH acidotic or alkalotic? Step 2- middle name- which sub-parameter matches the pH.- if PaCO2 matches then its "respiratory" as middle name and if HCO3 matches then the middle name is "metabolic". Step 3- ID level of compensation- acute (if pH and one sub-parameter match and the other sub-parameter is NORMAL), Mixed (all parameters either acidic or alkalotic), Partially compensated (if 3 No Rule present), and Fully compensation (if pH is normal and both sub-parameters are abnormal).

18. (**C**) With this patient, the lower temperature will shift the oxyhemoglobin disassociation curve to the left, along with a high affinity (stickiness) for oxygen by the red blood cell. This results in decreased release of a oxygen once the red blood cell is passing the tissues. This means that the RBC oxygen saturation is high, but oxygen is just not released from the red blood cell at the level of the tissues, therefore the tissues become hypoxic, acidic, and can die. Slurring does not happen on the QRS because of cold temperatures- Osbourne

waves do. Hyportension just does not occur because it's cold, and DIC does not occur just because a patient is entrapped.

19. (**B**) The oxyhemoglobin disassociation curve speaks to the affinity, or stickiness, of oxygen to the red blood cell. It does not discuss oxygen supply or demand. The real question here is it a left or a right shift. Remember that increased CO2 (as well as increased acid, temperature, & DPG) indicate a shift to the right.

20. (**D**) Reversing the I:E ratio will put the patient and maximal PEEP. This will help to maximize their oxygenation ability. Increasing the minute ventilation will not help, and increasing the tidal volume will essentially increase the minute ventilation, so these two is your selections are incorrect. Reducing PEEP will worsen oxygenation, so it is an incorrect answer is well.

21. (**A**) Partially compensated respiratory acidosis. Step 1- last name- is pH acidotic or alkalotic? Step 2- middle name- which sub-parameter matches the pH.- if PaCO2 matches then its "respiratory" as middle name and if HCO3 matches then the middle name is "metabolic". Step 3- ID level of compensation- acute (if pH and one sub-parameter match and the other sub-parameter is NORMAL), Mixed (all parameters either acidic or alkalotic), Partially compensated (if 3 No Rule present), and Fully compensation (if pH is normal and both sub-parameters are abnormal).

22. (**B**) Acute metabolic acidosis. Step 1- last name- is pH acidotic or alkalotic? Step 2- middle name- which sub-

parameter matches the pH.- if PaCO2 matches then its "respiratory" as middle name and if HCO3 matches then the middle name is "metabolic". Step 3- ID level of compensation- acute (if pH and one sub-parameter match and the other sub-parameter is NORMAL), Mixed (all parameters either acidic or alkalotic), Partially compensated (if 3 No Rule present), and Fully compensation (if pH is normal and both sub-parameters are abnormal).

23. **(C)** Step 1- last name- is pH acidotic or alkalotic? Step 2- middle name- which sub-parameter matches the pH.- if PaCO2 matches then its "respiratory" as middle name and if HCO3 matches then the middle name is "metabolic". Step 3- ID level of compensation- acute (if pH and one sub-parameter match and the other sub-parameter is NORMAL), Mixed (all parameters either acidic or alkalotic), Partially compensated (if 3 No Rule present), and Fully compensation (if pH is normal and both sub-parameters are abnormal).

24. **(C)** Fully compensated respiratory acidosis. This patient is overbreathing the vent (note her f is more than the set rate of 12) so they have blown off a lot of EtCO2 (28 mmHg). To fix this problem we need to sedate the patient which will reduce the frequency, and thus minute ventilation). This will in turn allow the EtCO2 to build back up. Increasing the RR to match the f is a practice that should never enter your mind. All that does is cover up the issue.

25. (B) PEEP will cause 2 different therapeutic phenomenons: it will increase alveolar surface area, and

it will thin the alveolar membrane. Both of these mechanisms will improve oxygenation.

26. (**D**) This patient is overbreathing the vent (note her f is more than the set rate of 15) so they have blown off a lot of EtCO2 (32 mmHg). To fix this problem we need to sedate the patient which will reduce the frequency, and thus minute ventilation). This will in turn allow the EtCO2 to build back up. Increasing the RR to match the f is a practice that should never enter your mind. All that does is cover up the issue.

27. This mode allows for spontaneous breaths. Some spontaneous breaths are allowed to happen unassisted, and some are assisted (these assisted breaths are assisting the patient's effort with pressure support). This mode does <u>not</u> synchronize to the patient with **EACH** breath, so that option is wrong- it only synchronizes the First breath in each breath cycle. It also doesn't require a paralytic nor does it automatically increase PEEP, so both those answers are wrong.

28. (**A**) This patient has an increased EtCO2 (52 mmHg) and to correct this problem we need to increase his minute ventilation. We could either increase RR or increase TV. There is no option to increase RR, but there is an option to increase TV, therefore, it is the correct answer.

29. (**D**) PEEP can reduce the Vte per breath. When you add PEEP you are actually asking the ventilator to breath stack some PEEP, which takes away from available lung real estate used to ventilate. Therefore, as you increase PEEP, you move LESS minute ventilation, and thus your

EtCO2 will elevate. So, you actually decrease the VE (minute ventilation) when you add PEEP.

30. (**B**) The verbal shorthand "17/5" is telling you that the pressure control (PC) is set at 17 and the PEEP is set at 5. You add these numbers together to get 22, so the PIP is 22. The ventilator is set to deliver 17 cmH2O into the patients lungs which is onto of the 5 cmH2O of PEEP that was left over from the last breath for a total of 22 cmH2O. Normal I:E is 1:2, so the I:E option is incorrect. We do not have the information to know the minute ventilation, so that option is also wrong.

31. (**B**) PEEP will cause 2 different therapeutic phenomenons: it will increase alveolar membrane surface area, and it will thin the alveolar membrane. Both of these mechanisms will improve oxygenation.

8 TOXICOLOGY

Questions

1. Several high school students develop altered mental status, hypotension, cherry red skin, and hyperthermia. They were all in the same classroom and they all fell ill at the same time. Which of the following conditions is most likely the cause?

    A. Carbon monoxide toxicity
    B. Amphetamine toxicity
    C. Methanol toxicity
    D. Serotonin syndrome

2. Your patient has ingested a handful of pills. The pill bottle reads, "Meperidine". Which of the following signs and symptoms would you anticipate in this patient?

    A. Salivation, lacrimation, and urinary issues
    B. Psychosis, hot/ flushed skin, pupil dilation
    C. Sedation, respiratory depression, myosis
    D. Tachycardia, hypertension, and agitation

3. You are treating a patient who has experienced a house fire and presents with flushed skin, dilated pupils, and an altered mental status. Reportedly he set the fire and took a bottle of pills. Which of the following substances is high on your differential diagnosis?

   A. Demerol OD
   B. Atropine OD
   C. Alcohol OD
   D. Elavil OD

4. A factory worker presents with severe drooling and tearing, and reports he has had very watery diarrhea that all began about an hour ago while at work. Which of the following treatment regimens is most appropriate in this patient?

   A. Atropine and oxygen
   B. 2-PAM and a benzo
   C. Activated charcoal
   D. RSI and intubation

5. While at a standby for a house fire, you get called over near the house to treat a firefighter. The patient has an altered mental status, bright red skin, and a pulse oximetry of 100%. Which of the following is the most appropriate action?

   A. RSI, intubate, and BVM the patient
   B. Admin high flow O2 immediately
   C. Deliver atropine and 2 PAM via IV
   D. Get the patient away from house

6. You are handed a bottle of pills that your patient took. You look up the name on the bottle; it is amitriptyline. Which of the following signs and symptoms would you most likely find in this patient?

   A. Drooling and copious diarrhea
   B. Mydriasis and hyperthermia
   C. Rhabdomyolysis and seizure
   D. Severe respiratory depression

7. Examine the ECG tracing below. This is from a patient you suspect has ingested a handful of pills in an attempt to commit suicide. Which of the following is the patient most likely suffering from?

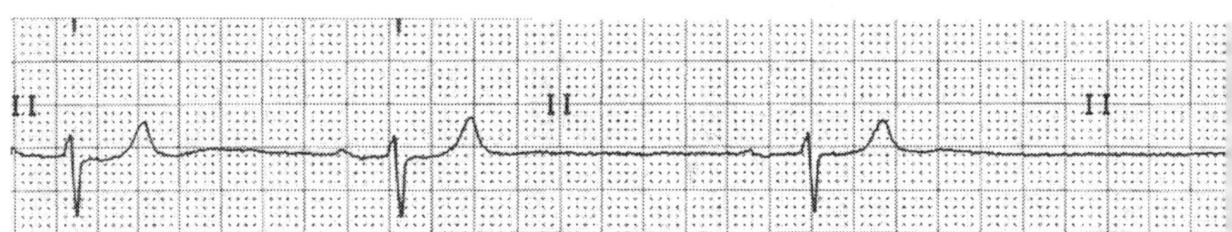

   A. Beta blocker OD
   B. Serotonin RI OD
   C. Tylenol overdose
   D. TCA overdose

8. Review the ECG below. This patient is an elderly woman with multiple co- morbid conditions who presented to the ER tonight with nausea and omitting and a decreasing mental status. Which of the following conditions is most likely occurring?

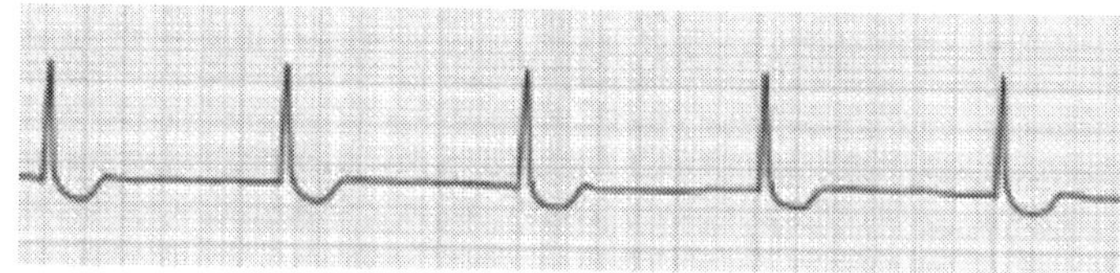

A. Cardiac glycoside toxicity
B. Acetaminophen toxicity
C. TCA/ Na blocker toxicity
D. Organophosphate toxicity

9. Your patient has been treated for 3 days for an acetaminophen OD. The medical staff reports (+) hepatomegaly, (+) coagulopathy, and severe jaundice. What phase of acetaminophen toxicity is the patient experiencing?

A. Phase I
B. Phase II
C. Phase III
D. Phase IV

10. Examine the ECG tracing below. What most likely will the antidote for this be?

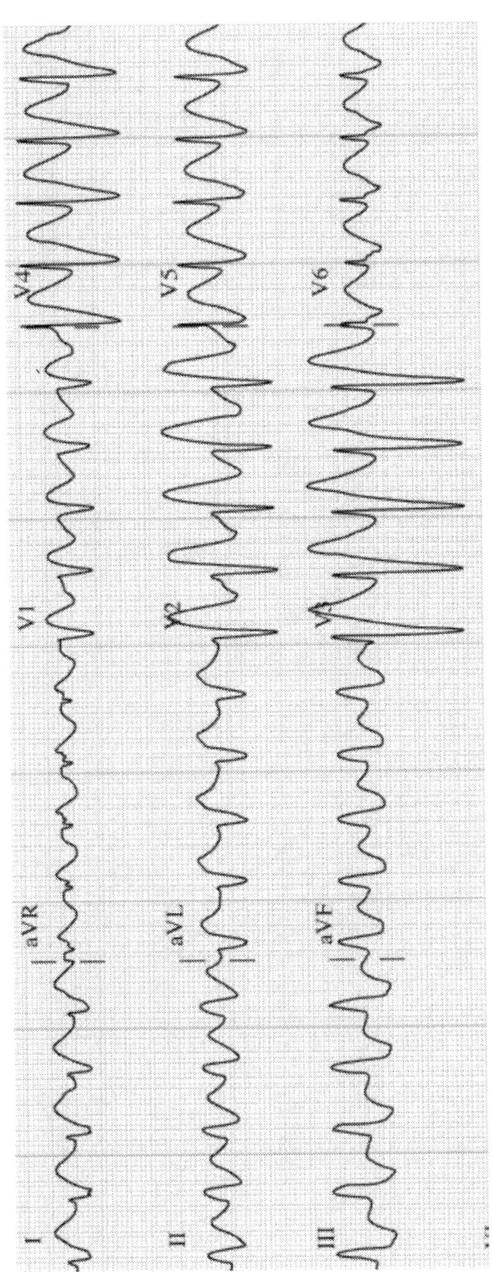

A. Physostigmine
B. 50g Glycogen
C. 1mg SQ epi
D. Ca gluconate

Answers

1. **(A)** The cherry red skin is a dead giveaway that these symptoms all point together to carbon monoxide poisoning. The underlying issue is a bad furnace where carbon monoxide is being produced and effecting all the kids of a classroom.

2. **(C)** These are the signs and symptoms of opioid intoxication and meperidine is the opioid Demerol.

3. **(D)** This patient fits the profile for 2 conditions: TCA OD and CO poisoning. A big red flag is the flushed skin. Now, the question didn't read "cherry red skin" but flushed skin should still drive you to put CO poisoning high on your differential. CO wasn't even an answer selection. The answer here is TCA overdose/ intoxication: Mad as a hatter (agitated), Red as a beet (flushed skin), and blind as a bat (pupil dilation). Making this even more complicated is you have to know that Elavil is a specific type of a TCA.

4. **(A)** These are one of those questions that makes you decide on a partial treatment. Know that these are out there. To figure this question out, you'll have to identify answer selections with partially correct information. In this case the only 2 are atropine/ oxygen and 2-PAM/ benzo. Ideally, you'd treat this patient with 2 PAM and atropine. So, look for the answer selections that have a piece of information that isn't correct. Oxygen would be treated with all ODs, but a benzo isn't necessary here. Therefore, the answer is atropine and oxygen.

5. **(D)** This patient is suffering from carbon monoxide poisoning. You could suffer the same fate if you do not first get away from the house. This is a common question set- up in toxicology because educators want you to always remember to take care of yourself first.

6. **(B)** This patient is experiencing a TCA overdose and amitriptyline is Elavil, which is a TCA. Blind as a bad (mydriasis- which is dilated pupils) and Hot as a hare (hyperthermia).

7. **(A)** This patient is experiencing a beta blocker OD as evidenced by the 1st degree heart block with sinus bradycardia. There isn't any characteristic ECG findings for serotonin and Tylenol. TCA overdoses display right axis deviation and a widening QRS.

8. **(A)** This ECG is displaying the ladle sign, therefore, this is suggestive of a digitalis, which is a cardiac glycoside.

9. **(C)** Remember the signs and symptoms of these phases. Phase III: 72-96 hours; oliguria, hepatomegaly, coagulopathy, liver failure.

10. **(A)** This is a TCA OD ECG tracing, therefore, the antidote would be Physostigmine. Notice the wide QRS and right axis deviation.

9 OBSTETRICS

Questions

1. You receive a report on your female patient. The patient is G3/P2/A1. What does this tell us?

   A. 3 abortions have occurred
   B. The patient delivered 3 times
   C. Currently, the patient is pregnant
   D. There is very high risk of PIH

2. Describe the variability in the provided tracing.

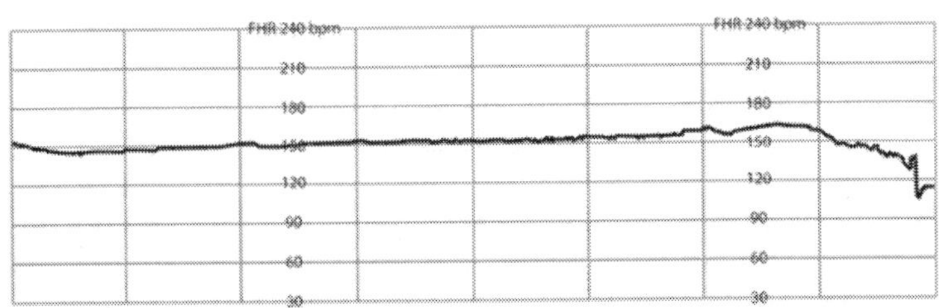

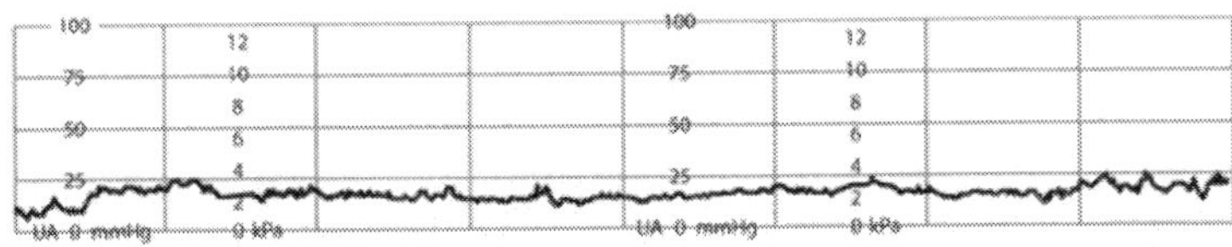

A. Marked Variability
B. Moderate Variability
C. Normal variability
D. Poor variability

3. In the provided toco monitor tracing, how far apart are the patient's contractions?

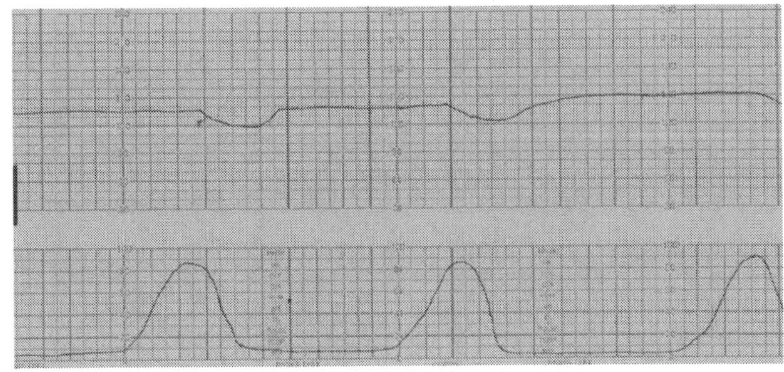

A. 6.5 minutes apart
B. 3.5 minutes apart
C. 9.5 minutes apart
D. 1.5 minutes apart

4. Your pregnant patient is complaining of fatigue and malaise. Her first pregnancy resulted in gestational diabetes. She currently is presenting with these vital signs: HR 98, RR 22, BP 162/102, and pulse oximetry of 94%. Paired with this information, which of the following findings is consistent with PIH?

   A. 125 mg/dL of protein in urine; (+) platelets < 400
   B. 455 mg/dL of protein in urine; (+) peripheral edema
   C. (+) platelets less than 400; (+) peripheral edema
   D. High liver enzymes; (+) platelets of less than 100

5. Describe the variability in the provided tracing.

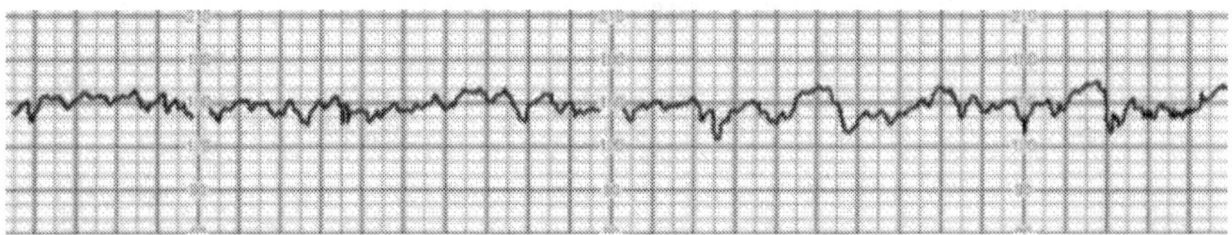

   A. Poor variability
   B. Moderate Variability
   C. Normal variability
   D. Marked Variability

6. Your patient is in labor and you are transporting them to a hospital with better OB receiving capabilities. Examine the fetal monitor tracing below and choose the most likely pathophysiology present.

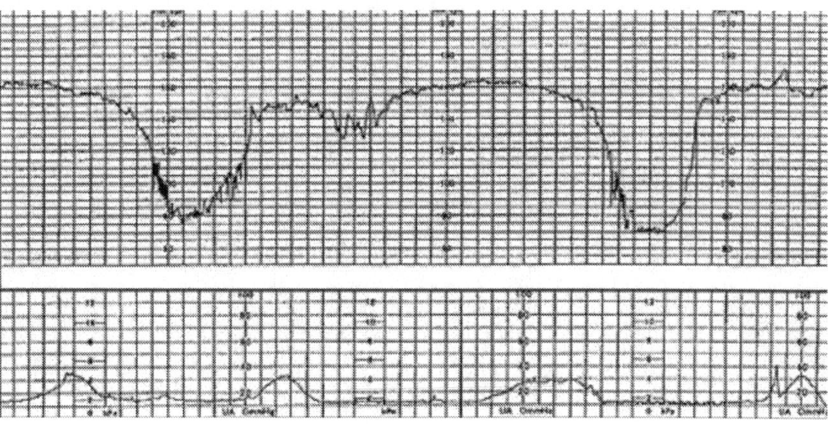

A. Significant fetal hypoxia
B. Severe fetal alkalosis
C. An uterine Rupture
D. A placental previa

7. You are treating a patient in labor. She is 38 weeks gestation. Upon the last contraction, you notice crowning. After the contraction, the infants head was retracted back into the vagina. This occurs with the next 2 contractions without change. What treatment should immediately execute?

A. Preform an episiotomy
B. McRobert's maneuver
C. Preform Valsalva
D. Breech birth maneuver

8. A patient presents with a history of endometriosis. She is currently experiencing abdominal pain and vaginal bleeding. She is 26 years old. What needs to first be ruled out?

   A. Ruptured ovarian cyst
   B. Pelvic inflammatory disease
   C. Toxic shock syndrome
   D. An ectopic pregnancy

9. You look down at the fetal monitor strip and notice the below tracing. What is causing this particular pattern on the tracing?

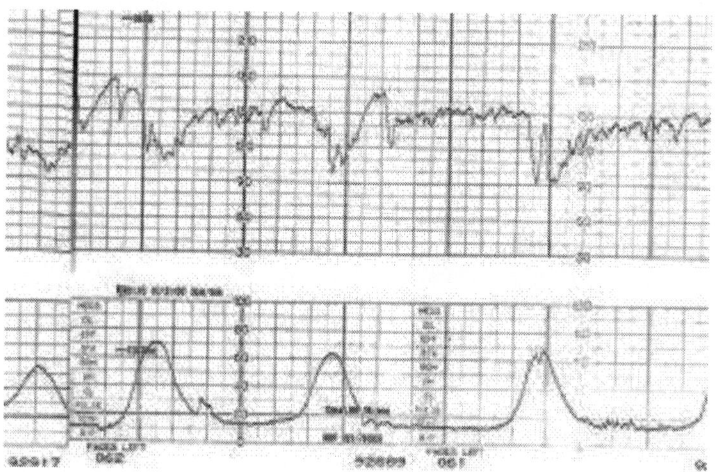

   A. Placental previa
   B. Uterine Rupture
   C. Cord compression
   D. Preeclampsia

10. You are en route to transport a pregnant patient who currently presents with G1,P0,A0, 34 weeks gestation, contractions are 11 minutes apart with maximal intensity with each and every contraction. Which of the following would be most appropriate in this case?

A. The patient has birthed 1 child already
B. Magnesium sulfate needs to be administered
C. Execute the Wood's corkscrew maneuver
D. Delivery is imminent, so prepare to deliver.

11. You are assessing your pregnant patient and note the following toco tracing. From this tracing, which of the following is correct regarding the condition of the fetus?

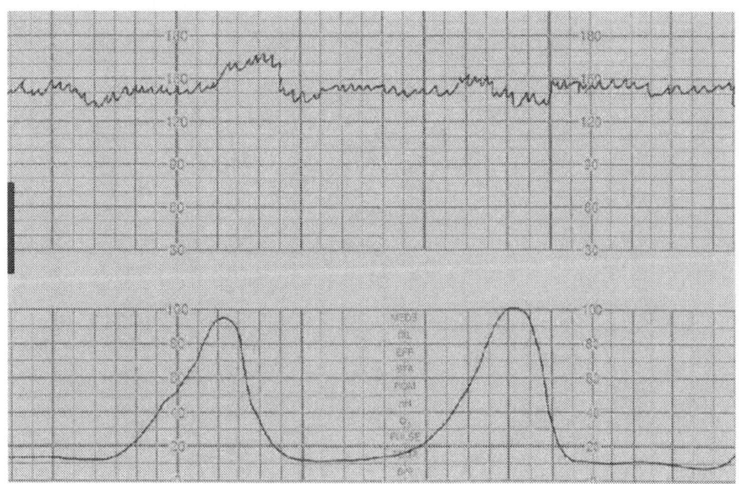

A. The fetus is in acidosis
B. Acute cord compression
C. This is a healthy fetus
D. Acute abruptio placenta

12. Describe the variability in the above tracing.

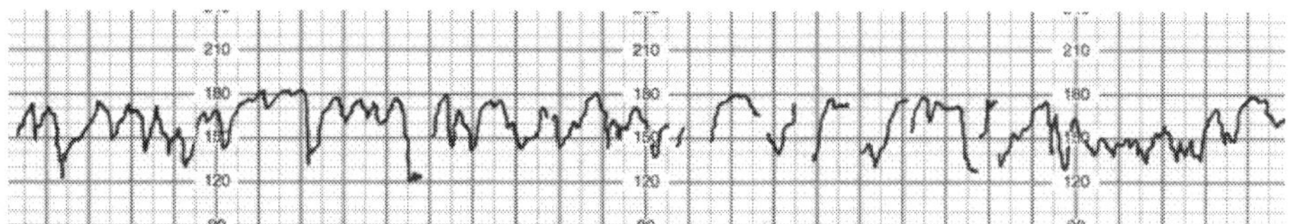

A. Marked Variability
B. Moderate Variability
C. Normal variability
D. Poor variability

13. You notice on your fetal monitoring equipment that your patient's fetus is experiencing late decelerations as well as poor variability. You recognize these two findings as being suggestive of which of the following?

A. Fetal movement
B. Strong fetal stability
C. Ominous findings
D. Normal assessment

14. You receive a report from the sending facility that a pregnant patient has received Rhogam. From this, what do we know about the mother and the child?

A. Mom (Rh+) and fetus (Rh-), this is the patient's first pregnancy
B. Mom (Rh-) and fetus (Rh+), the patient has been pregnant before
C. Mom (Rh-) and fetus (Rh-), this is the patient's first pregnancy
D. Mom (Rh+) and fetus (Rh+), the patient has been pregnant before

15. You're pregnant patient is experiencing labor. The sending nurse reports that your patient is at a +5 station and fully dilated. What does this tell you?

A. Delivery likely to occur within minutes
B. There are hours before delivery will occur
C. The patient could deliver within 60 minutes
D. Not enough information to make decision

Answers

1. (**C**) Gradiva: total number of all pregnancies (including the current pregnancy); Para: total number of deliveries after 20 weeks gestation; Abortions- number of abortions. Therefore, this patient is currently pregnant, has been pregnant 3 times, delivered twice and has had 1 abortion.

2. (**D**) The variability reflects the baby's fight or flight response (sympathetic response). A healthy and oxygenated fetus will have MODERATE variability and accelerations. A fetus who is being starved of oxygen for any reason will present with low (aka poor) variability and later decelerations. Moderate variability looks like course ventricular fibrillation while poor variability looks like asystole. In this case, the correct answer is poor variability.

3. (**B**) Each small box represents 10 seconds and there is 6 small boxes before a bold line occurs. Therefore, each bold line represents a minute. The contractions here are 3.5 minutes apart.

4. (**B**) The classic triad of high blood pressure, proteinuria, and edema strongly indicates PIH, thus is the correct answer of this question.

5. (**A**) The variability reflects the baby's fight or flight response (sympathetic response). A healthy and oxygenated fetus will have MODERATE variability and accelerations. A fetus who is being starved of oxygen for

any reason will present with low (aka poor) variability and later decelerations. Moderate variability looks like course ventricular fibrillation while poor variability looks like asystole. In this case, the correct answer is moderate variability.

6. (**A**) A late deceleration is an indication of prolonged fetal hypoxia and possible acidosis. You are behind the oxygen 8- ball in these cases and need to act quickly to correct the fetal hypoxia. While these other conditions can cause fetal hypoxia, a late deceleration is SPECIFIC to fetal hypoxia of any etiology, therefore, "significant fetal hypoxia" is the correct answer.

7. (**B**) Turtle sign indicates shoulder dystocia. At this point, the McRobert's maneuver should be performed which involves quickly flexing the legs against the patient's abdomen- this causes the birth canal to slightly widen. The Woods corkscrew maneuver should be performed next which involves turning the fetus by inserting your hands into the vagina, grasping its shoulders and spinning the baby 180 degrees. The fetus naturally corkscrews as it travels through the birth canal and sometimes gets a shoulder caught on the pubic bone (shoulder dystocia). By turning the baby, you mimic this corkscrew action which can free up the baby's shoulder. Another option is to pull out the baby's arm which reduces the baby's width and thus allowing delivery.

8. (**D**) The ectopic pregnancy should be ruled out first because it can cause significant bleeding and death.

9. (**C**) This Tracing exhibits 3 decelerations that are VARIABLE

because they differ in magnitude (they are all different depths and widths). This indicates the umbilical cord is being compressed.

10. (**D**) Remember that signs of imminent labor include contractions are 5-7 minutes apart over the period of an hour; all contractions have the same, or very similar, intensity; 100% effaced and fully dilated- there are all signs of imminent delivery, so you should prepare your equipment for delivery. It isn't the best idea to put this patient in your aircraft. Deliver, then arrange/ discuss transport with medical direction.

11. (**C**) The tracing exhibits accelerations, which are ONLY possible in a well oxygenated, and non-acidotic, fetus. Therefore, the answer here is a "healthy fetus".

12. (**B**) This looks like course ventricular fibrillation, therefore, it is MODERATE variability.

13. (**C**) One of the worst tracings possible for a fetus is a persistent decelerations with poor variability. This means the baby is extremely tired and will not be able to continue fighting acidosis. This is very OMINOUS. Act quickly to correct or have the MD perform a C-section.

14. (**B**) During a Rh negative mom's first pregnancy with an Rh positive fetus, blood mixing during delivery sensitizes mom to the Rh positive protein on the baby's RBCs. Subsequent pregnancies with a Rh positive baby (and Rh negative mom) can lead to mom's blood attacking the Rh positive baby's blood. In subsequent pregnancies, the mother may receive Rhogam to prevent mom's blood from attacking the baby's blood.

15. (**A**) Remember that station is a way to describe where the child is in the birth canal. A positive number means the child is coming closer to the vaginal opening, while a negative number means they have not traveled very far from the uterus. Therefore, a positive number means that labor has begun and that fetus is moving towards delivery. A station of +5 means that crowning probably is occurring, so delivery is likely to occur very quickly.

10 NEONATOLOGY

Questions

1. Your patient was born 5 minutes ago and required mechanical ventilation. The patient is being ventilated via BVM at a rate of 29 and with room air. Which of the following actions is most appropriate in this case?

   A. Target an SpO2 of 80-85%
   B. Increase the RR to 35/ min
   C. Apply BVM to 100% oxygen
   D. Administer a prostaglandin

2. Which of the following pathophysiologies is considered a cyanotic condition?

   A. VSD
   B. ASD
   C. TOF
   D. PDA

3. Your 2.5kg neonatal patient is failing to respond to additional stimulation and positive pressure ventilation. You decide to intubate the patient. Which of the following treatment regimens is most appropriate for this patient?

   A. 2.5mm tube at 6cm at the lip
   B. 3.5mm tube at 8.5cm at the lip
   C. 3.0mm tube at 7cm at the lip
   D. 4.0mm tube at 10cm at the lip

4. You are transporting a neonate patient who blinks their eyes every few seconds and has eye deviation between the blinking. Which of the following treatment is most appropriate and this patient?

   A. Administer surfactant
   B. Admin indomethicin
   C. Admin prostaglandin
   D. Administer ativan

5. You're treating your neonate patient for hypotension that you suspect is from sepsis. Your patient weighs 7 pounds. Which of the following management actions is appropriate for this patient?

   A. 26 cc over 1 minute
   B. 36 cc over 10 minutes
   C. 22 cc over via bolus
   D. 32 cc over 5 minutes

6. Your neonatal patient has pale extremities and is without brachial pulses. The patient ways 11 pounds. Following your initial fluid Bolus, what is an appropriate maintenance rate for this patient?
   A. 9 cc/hr
   B. 20 cc/hr
   C. 42 cc/hr
   D. 16 cc/hr

7. You are responding to a 9 day old infant who was sent home 2 days after delivery. The patient has not been feeding well and exhibits difficulty breathing. Which of the following is true regarding management of this patient?

   A. 20 cc/kg bolus will be needed on this patient
   B. The umbilical vein for venous access is off limits
   C. D10 fluid resuscitation to prevent hypoglycemia
   D. Avoid scalp veins since they can cause emboli

8. It is reported to you that your newborn patient presents with pulmonary stenosis, a high riding aorta, and a hypertrophic right ventricle. Which of the following management actions is most appropriate?

   A. Tracheal Suctioning
   B. Prostaglandins
   C. Surfactant dosing
   D. High flow oxygen

9. You have medical control orders to administer prostaglandins to close your patient's PDA. The patient ways 11 pounds. Which of the following the correct dosage for PGE1 for this patient?

   A. 1.0 mcg/kg/min
   B. 2.0 mcg/min
   C. 0.4 mcg/min
   D. 1.5 mcg/kg/min

10. A primie infant delivered tonight is approximately 7 weeks premature and presents with respiratory difficulty. Which of the following interventions are most appropriate in this case?

    A. Administer versed
    B. Administer surfactant
    C. Admin indomethicin
    D. Admin prostaglandin

Answers

1. (**A**) During the fifth minute of life, pre ductal pulse oximetry should be between 80 to 85%. This case our patient is at 90%. It is prudent to target 80 to 85% pulse oximetry.

2. (**C**) TOF is Tetralogy of Fallot and is characterized by several conditions which lead to a right to left shunting of blood. VSD, ASD, and PDA are all acyanotic lesions.

3. (**B**) This patient is 2.5kg, so by NRP requires a 3.5mm size endotracheal tube. The depth of the tube can be estimated by the KG + 6, again, as per NRP. A 33 week old kid will weigh typically between 1-2 kg (Remember: gestational ago 28 weeks- up to 1kg; 28-34 weeks- 1-2 kg; 34-38 weeks- 2-3 kg; above 38 weeks-above 3kg. Therefore, this patient requires 3.0mm and secured at 9cm at the lip.

4. (**D**) This patient is having a seizure. Signs and symptoms of a seizure in a neonate is as follows: eye deviation; blinking; pedaling movements of the legs; tonic extension of the extremities; flexion of extremities; convulsions. Therefore the base and as a peeve would be appropriate in this case to stop the seizure.

5. (**D**) The dosage for volume expansion and a due date is 10 cc/kg. This patient ways 7 pounds, which is equivalent to 3.18 kilograms. Therefore the dosage should be approximately 32 cc of normal saline or blood. This should be given over 5 or 10 minutes (slowly). Remember, neonatal veins are very fragile, and pushing rapidly could

damage their vessels. This patient should receive 32 cc over 5-10 minutes.

6. (**B**) The patient's initial maintenance rate in this case should be 20 cc/hour. The patient ways 11 pounds, which is the equivalent of 5 kg. Using the 4/2/1 method of calculating maintenance rates, the first 5 kilograms is multiplied by four, yielding 20 cc/hr.

7. (**B**) The umbilical vein should not be access after 7 days.

8. (**B**) With the provided pathophysiology, your patient is presented with Tetralogy of Fallot. In this case, you should **avoid** high flow oxygen which could cause the ductus arteriosus to close. In these patients the patent ductus arteriosus is the one thing keeping oxygenated blood being introduced into the systemic circulation. High oxygen or the drug indomethicin will close the PDA which can result in death of your patient. Prostaglandins will keep the PDA open, so it is the appropriate action.

9. (**C**) Prostaglandin is administered 0.1 mcg/kg/min. The patient ways 9 pounds, which is the equivalent of 4.09 kg. Therefore, 0.1 mcg/kg/min multiplied by the patient's weight in kilograms yields 0.4 mg/min.

10. (**B**) Premature infants they need surfactant. You can be proactive by simply identifying the gestational age of the patient and then anticipating some of the problems that can be encountered with premature infants- one of which is respiratory distress syndrome from inadequate surfactant.

11 PEDIATRICS

Questions

1. You are transporting a pediatric patient with an underdeveloped left ventricle and poorly formed ascending aorta. What general management plan is most appropriate with this patient?

   A. Measure O2 sats from pre and post ductal sites
   B. Apply high flow O2 via non-rebreather mask
   C. Immediately intubate the patient apply vent
   D. Administer a fluid bolus of 10 cc/kg of NS

2. An 8kg infant presents weak and poorly reactive to their environment and with sunken fontanels. The mother reports the patient hasn't been feeding well. Which the following the most appropriate management for this patient?

   A. 240 cc/kg NS
   B. 80 cc/kg NS
   C. 160 cc/kg LR
   D. 320 cc/kg LR

3. You are told your pediatric patient has a ventricular septal defect. Which of the following is true regusrding it's management?

   A. It is safe to administer oxygen
   B. Avoid high flow oxygen admin
   C. Monitor pre/post ductal O2 sats
   D. Keep O2 sats between 70-80%

4. Your pediatric patient needs requires intubation. Which of the following formulas would you use to calculate the endotracheal tube size?

   A. (Age + 4)/16
   B. (Age x 2) + 8
   C. 4 + (4/Age)
   D. (Age/4) + 4

5. An 18 month old is to be transfered to a peditric center. They currently present with inspiratory retractions, a loud scratcy cough, and stridor. Which of the following conditions is the child most likely suffered from?

   A. Bronchiolitis
   B. Epiglotitis
   C. (+) Croup
   D. (+) FBAO

6. A 15 month old child is being administered dopamine. The 12 kg child is receiving a pediatric concentration of dopamine

(800mg/ 250cc). Which of the following flow rates is achieving an alpha dose of dopamine?

A. 0.5 cc/hr
B. 1.4 cc/hr
C. 2.7 cc/hr
D. 4.5 cc/hr

7. A 7-year-old male with anemia presents with severe right upper quadrant abdominal pain, low oxygen saturation, and priapism. These signs and symptoms suggest which presentation?

A. Appendicitis
B. Diabetes Mellitus
C. Hemorrhaging
D. Sickle cell crisis

8. Your 12 month old patient is presenting with shortness of breath, fever, and wheezes. Which of the following conditions is the child most likely suffered from?

A. Bronchiolitis
B. Epiglotitis
C. (+) Croup
D. (+) FBAO

9. Upon assessemnt of your infant patient, you assess for a Babinski reflex. Which of the following is true reguarding this assessment?

A. It's executed by striking toes to heel
B. Flexion of the big toe is a positive sign
C. Fanning of the toes is a normal finding
D. It's abnormal in infants but not in adults

10. Your pediatric patient presents with hypoglycemia and is 11kg infant. You are currently mixing a 30 cc syringe of dextrose 10%. How would you mix at the D10 concentration?

A. Take 22 cc from D50 and mix with 6cc NS
B. Mix 11grams of dextrose in 24 cc of 0.9 NS
C. Take 6 cc from D50 and mix with 24 cc NS
D. Mix 11 grams of dextrose in 27 cc of 0.9 NS

11. Your pediatric patient has a HA. Upon evaluation while lying on the exam table, he bends hihip and knees (beinds knees towards the chest) when you flex their neck (head to chest motion). Which of the following signs does this represent?

A. SIDS sign
B. Brudzinski sign
C. Kernig sign
D. Concussion sign

12. Your patient is a 3 year old with temperature of 102.3 F following aspiration 2 days ago. Currently the patient presents with warm flushed skin, tachycardia, and irritability. Which of the following conditions is indicated?

A. Hypovolemic shock
B. Neurogenic shock
C. Shock from sepsis
D. Cardiagenic shock

13. A pediatric patient with RSV has the following vital signs: BP 92/42, HR 138, pulse oximetry 86% and EtCO2 of 41. The ventilator is currently set at SIMV RR 36, PC 15, I:E 1:2, FiO2 1.0, Vte 42 , PEEP 5, PIP 20, AutoPEEP is 0. Which of the following would be the most appropriate action?

A. Reduce RR 28
B. Reverse the I:E
C. Decrease PC 13
D. Increase PEEP 7

14. A 20 month old patient presents with rapidly developing shortness of breath, fever, and drooling. Which of the following conditions is the child most likely suffered from?

A. Bronchiolitis
B. Epiglotitis
C. (+) Croup
D. (+) FBAO

15. A febrile 5 month old presents with a tapering of the upper trachea on a frontal chest x-ray. Which of the following conditions is your patient likely experiencing?

A. (+) Croup
B. Epiglottitis
C. (+) FBAO
D. Pneumonia

16. Your transporting a 4 month old infant. This patient is experiencing a narrowing of the descending portion of the aorta resulting in a limited flow of blood to the lower part of the body. Which of the following treatments would be appropriate?

A. Provider high flow O2
B. Administer surfactant
C. Maintain MAP at 70
D. Give prostaglandin E1

Answers

1. (**A**) In hypopastic left heart syndrome, the left ventricle is poorly formed. Additionally, the mitral valve and the aortic valves fail to form. These patients rely on an open PDA and VSDs to deliver some oxygenated blood to the systemic circulation. KEEP THE PDA OPEN. In cyanotic neonates, transcutaneous oxygen saturation (ie, pulse oximetry) should be measured from preductal (right hand) and postductal sites (right or left foot). Oxygen saturation values are reduced with central cyanosis and usually normal with peripheral cyanosis. A difference in values at the two sites identifies patients with differential cyanosis. In patients with a right aortic arch, the preductal saturation should be measured in the left hand. The routine use of pulse oximetry to screen for neonatal critical cardiac disease has been shown to be an effective screening test and is discussed separately.

2. (**C**) This patient should be treated with an infusion of 20 CC's per kilo of isotonic crystalloid and a blood glucose determination. The history of prolonged vomiting and diarrhea suggest hypovolemia. Therefore this child must be treated with aggressive fluid resuscitation and reassessment.

3. (**D**) A ventricular septal defect (VSD) is a hole or a defect in the septum that divides the 2 lower chambers of the heart, resulting in communication between the ventricular cavities. A VSD may occur as a primary anomaly, with or without additional major associated cardiac defects. You do not need to avoid oxygen nor would you have to monitor pre/post ductal oxygen sats. You also would not have to keep the oxygen sats between 70-80%: 94-99% would be acceptable.

4. (**D**) When determining the size of an endotracheal tube in a

pediatric patient, there are a few different formulas. We offer these two formulas to calculate and a tracheal to a size: (AGE/4) + 4mm, or (Age + 16)/4. Therefore in this case the answer is (AGE/4) + 4mm.

5. (**C**) This child has croup. Foreign body airway obstruction is suspected of situations were a previously healthy, afebrile child rapidly develops signs and symptoms of respiratory distress. Epiglottitis is characterized by a rapid onset, high fever, and drooling. Bronchiolitis usually occurs in children under one years old and presents with wheezing. Therefore the answer to this question is croup.

6. (**B**) There is only one flow rate provided that would be toasting the patient with and the alpha range. [(1.4 cc/hr)(800mg x 1000mcg/mg)]/ (250cc)/(60cc/hr)/ (wt in KG, or 12) = 6 mcg/kg/min. Be sure to practice your drug calculations for these exams. **Take a look at my textbook, Calc Hero, for a systematic approach and practice for calculation infusion problems, including the ability to calculate backwards. Its much easier than you think.**

7. (**D**) Sickle cell crisis can cause vasoocclusive pain, stroke, anemia, AMI, renal infarction, PIH (if pregnant), and priapism. Ultimately, sickle cell crisis causes misshapen and hard RBCs that do not accept oxygen well.

8. (**A**) This child has Bronchiolitis. Foreign body airway obstruction is suspected of situations were a previously healthy, afebrile child rapidly develops signs and symptoms of respiratory distress. Epiglottitis is characterized by a rapid onset, high fever, and drooling. Bronchiolitis usually occurs in children under one years old and presents with wheezing. Therefore the answer to this question is croup.

9. (**C**) The Babinski reflex is obtained by stimulating the outside of

the sole of the foot, causing extension of the big toe while fanning the other toes. The examiner begins the stimulation at the heel and goes forward to the base of the toes. Most newborn babies and young infants are not neurologically mature, and they therefore show a Babinski reflex. A Babinski reflex in an older child or an adult is abnormal and is a sign of a problem in the brain or spinal cord.

10. (**C**) Remember a "percent" solution really means mix that percentage of drug with the reciprocal percentage of normal saline. In this case we need 3 g of dextrose into a 30cc syringe, because three is 10% of 30. Dextrose 50 is mixed 25 g in a 50 cc ampule (25 is half of 50, or 50%). This means that every cc of D50 contains 0.5g of dextrose. To get 3g, we need to remove 6cc from the D50 ampule and mix it with 24cc of normal saline. that gives us 3g in 30cc, or D10.

11. (**B**) Brudzinski's the sign is also seen in meningitis. It is characterized by the flexion of the neck that usually causes flexion of the hip and knees. Kernig's sign is a sign seen with meningitis patients and is characterized by the inability to complete leaks and a leg when sitting or lying down.

12. (**C**) Tachycardia with bounding pulses; warm, flushed skin, delayed capillary refill, inherent ability are all likely findings in the pediatric patient with early septic shock (aka warm shock). The cool phase of septic shock occurs when cardiac output drops (measurable by cardiac output itself, or a lowering trend in the blood pressure) and the skin becomes cool to the touch.

13. (**D**) The only issue with the data provided is the low oxygen saturation, which can be fixed with increased FiO2 or PEEP. In this case the FiO2 is maxed out, therefore, increase PEEP to correct the low pulse oximetry.

14. (**B**) This child has Epiglottitis. Foreign body airway obstruction is

suspected of situations were a previously healthy, afebrile child rapidly develops signs and symptoms of respiratory distress. Epiglottitis is characterized by a rapid onset, high fever, and drooling. Bronchiolitis usually occurs in children under one years old and presents with wheezing. Therefore the answer to this question is croup.

15. (**A**) Croup is a viral infection of the upper airway that can affect the larynx, trachea, and bronchi; known for its 'barking cough'. It presents with low grade fever; 'barking cough'; mild distress; stridor; and STEEPLE SIGN on X-ray.

16. (**D**) This describes the condition called coarctation of the aorta and prostaglandin E1 is needed to maintain the patency of the ductus arteriosus. The dose is 0.025 to 0.05 mcg/kg per minute and increase as needed to a maximum dose of 0.1 mcg/kg per minute. High flow O2 would SHUT the PDA and worsen, if not kill, the patient. Surfactant is not indicated.

12 BURNS

Questions

1. Your patient has severe thermal burns to the neck, chest, abdomen, and back from being trapped in a vehicle that caught on fire. You now have them on the mechanical ventilator. The original PIP was 16 cmH2O and 20 minutes later it is 52 cmH2O. Which intervention may be indicated?

   A. Increase PEEP
   B. Needle chest
   C. Escharotomy
   D. BVM bagging

2. You arrive to transport a patient involved in a flash fire in a large cylindrical holding tank that he was cleaning. Your assessment reveals a patent airway, (+) breath sounds with wheezes in the distal airways. The patient is calm, but

in pain. They exhibit symmetrical chest rise and fall. What is the most appropriate next action?

A. Cricothyrotomy
B. BVM ventilations
C. Bronchodilator
D. Prepare for CPAP

3. Fluid resuscitation has begun for a 81kg patient with 21% partial thickness burns. The burn was 3 hours ago and the sending facility has infused 630cc LR. What does the astute critical care clinician recognize in reference to fluid resuscitation?

A. Inadequate- 100cc low
B. Adequate and appropriate
C. Inadequate- 200cc low
D. Not enough information

4. Fluid resuscitation has begun for a 100kg patient with 29% partial thickness burns. The burn was 3.5 hours ago and the sending facility has infused 1000cc LR. What does the astute critical care clinician recognize in reference to fluid resuscitation in this case?

A. Adequate and appropriate
B. Inadequate- about 750cc low
C. Inadequate- about 250cc low
D. Not enough information here

5. Your patient was involved in an industrial fire involving a textile warehouse. Their vitals are as follows: HR 118, RR 15, BP 119/70, SpO2 99%, and the skin is pink/ warm/ dry. Which of the following is the patient most likely experiencing?

   A. Stagnant hypoxia
   B. CO poisoning
   C. Hypovolemia
   D. Inhalation injury

6. Your patient was injured in an explosion resulting in a hemothorax. You discover the following lab values: Na 142, Ca 10, K 4.3, Glu 87, Cl 100, HCO3 23, BUN 12, H/H 8 and 18. What is the most appropriate action?

   A. Transfuse PRBCs
   B. Prepare to intubate
   C. Needle decompress
   D. Place a central line

7. Your adult patient has suffered thermal burns resulting in excessive partial and full thickness burns to the lower extremities. The patient's vitals are as follows: HR 112, BP 118/74, RR 22. The patient presents with strong radial pulses and diminished dorsalis pedis pulses bilaterally. What should immediately be done?

   A. Escharotomy
   B. BVM ventilation
   C. Apply dry sheets
   D. Intubation

8. You are transporting an electrical burn patient. Their vital signs are as follows: HR 101, RR 17, BP 124/82, SpO2 99%, EtCO2 42, temp 36.9C, Na 139, K 3.9, Cl 101, HCO3 22, BUN 16, Glu 102, Cr 0.9, UO 28cc/h, H/H 15 and 45. The patient weighs 72kg. What is the next most appropriate action?

   A. Prepare to intubate pt
   B. No changes are needed
   C. Prepare mag infusion
   D. Increase isotonic fluids

9. As you are reviewing the chart of the 85kg burn patient you are about to transport to a larger hospital, the RN reports the following: HR 87, RR 15, BP 141/82, SpO2 97%, EtCO2 44, temp 37C, Na 144, K 4.1, Cl 104, HCO3 24, BUN 13, Glu 97, Cr 0.8, UO 33cc/h, H/H 17 and 47. What is the next most appropriate action?

   A. Increase isotonic fluids
   B. Prepare to intubate pt
   C. No changes are needed
   D. Prepare mag infusion

10. Your patient was injured from being trapped in a house fire. Upon assessment, the patient presents with burns to the lips and hoarse voice. The patient has 15% third degree to his back as well. What condition are you most concerned about?

A. Compartment syndrome
B. Circumferential burn
C. Inhalation injury
D. Severe thermal burn

11. After experiencing a nearby explosion, your patient has suffered 25% BSA full and partial thickness burns to the front side of his body. What condition should be suspected?

A. Circumferential burn
B. Compartment syndrome
C. Tension pneumothorax
D. Inhalation injury

12. Your patient was recently rescued from a house fire. Upon looking into the lab report, you discover these values: Na 144, Ca 10, K 3.9, Glu 102, Cl 100, HCO3 27, SvO2 70, BUN 15, H/H 14 and 42. Does this patient exhibit signs of cyanide toxicity?

A. No- there is not a significant anion gap
B. No- cyanide isn't produced in fires
C. Yes- metabolic acidosis is present
D. Yes- the tachypnea alone indicates it

Answers

1. (**C**) The patient is severely burned to the chest and back, so circumferential burns are likely. The critical care clinician needs to be prepared for poor chest expansion due to these circumferential burns. This would cause peak inspiratory pressure to rise and alarm. If the high pressure is due to the hardening skin from the circumferential burn, then an escharotomy is indicated. BVM/ needle chest/increase PEEP- wrong because it would not fix the rigidity of the chest. The chest needs o be cut to allow for chest wall expansion.

2. (**C**) Wheezes indicates bronchodilation, so use bronchodilators to open them up. Don't rush to cut the neck here- try a less invasive therapy. BVM ventilations seem overkill here too because they are breathing calmly indicating they are not acutely hypoxic. CPAP could actually worsen bronchoconstriction.

3. (**B**) The consensus formula is (2cc x %BSA x KG), so in this case we get (2cc x 21 x 81) = 3402cc to be given in 24 hours. Half this total volume is 1701 and is to be given in the first 8 hours. (1725cc/8h = 212cc/h, so in 3 hours the patient should have received 637cc The patient has received the appropriate amount of fluid at this point.

4. (**C**) The consensus formula is (2cc x %BSA x KG), so in this case we get (2cc x 29 x 100) = 5800cc to be given in 24 hours. Half this total volume is 2900 and is to be given in

the first 8 hours. (2900cc/8h = 362cc/h, so in 3.5 hours the patient should have received 1268cc. They only received 1000cc,(1268-1000 = deficit of 268cc), therefore, the answer is "about 250 low".

5. (**B**) The HR and RR indicate the body is increasing efforts to push oxygen forward (a sign of hypoxia) but the skin is warm and pink (non- cyanotic). If you take these 2 pieces of information with the history of a house fire, then you have a situation consistent with CO poisoning. Stagnant hypoxia is when blood isn't moving forward like it should, there is nothing here to suggest an inhalation injury, and BP is normal, so hypovolemia is unlikely.

6. (**A**) The H/H is telltale here, and specifically the hemoglobin (its 8 here and hematocrit is 18), therefore a transfusion is necessary. We have no information here to indicate intubation because we don't know mental or hemodynamic status. Needle decompression won't correct a hemothorax- chest tubes are needed. A central line is not an absolute in this case, sure t would help, but the correct answer is to transfuse some RBCs.

7. (**A**) The loss of pedal pulses are key in this case and indicates the arterial blood supply to the feet are compromised by the circumferential burn. While most agencies do not allow for extremity escharotomy, some do. If you work for an agency that does not allow, then know it is time for rapid transport and quick (but safe) transition to and from the aircraft/ambulance to the destination.

8. (**D**) The key here is the low urine output (UO) of 28cc/hr. Adequate fluid resuscitation in a burn patient would be indicated by a UO of 0.5-1cc/kg/min. In this case, 72kg x 0.5cc/hr = 36cc/h. It is reported that the patient has a UO of 28cc/hr, or a deficit of 8cc/hr, therefore, we need to increase the fluids to meet this minimum UO.

9. (**C**) The key here is the low urine output (UO) of 33cc/hr. Adequate fluid resuscitation in a burn patient would be indicated by a UO of 0.5-1cc/kg/min. In this case, 65kg x 0.5cc/hr = 32.5cc/h. It is reported that the patient has a UO of 33cc/hr. Additionally, all other values are normal, therefore, no changes are needed.

10. (**C**) The key here is the burned lips and hoarse voice in a patient who was burned. This indicates an inhalation injury, and thus the patient should be intubated right away.

11. (**D**) The key here is the explosion. This indicates an inhalation injury is potentially present, and thus the continued assessment should be looking for those tell-tale findings indicating inhalation injury: facial burns/ stridor/ hoarse voice/ carbon deposits around airway circumferential neck burns/ soot around nose.

12. (**A**) Remember, air hunger (tachypnea- not present) with metabolic acidosis indicates cyanide poisoning/ toxicity, so when given the components of the anion gap, be sure to calculate it. In this case, (139 + 4.1) - (107 + 27) = 9.1. Since the anion gap is < 16, then no anion gap is evident and evidence for cyanide poisoning is weak. If SvO2 was high, then that is also evidence of poor O2 uptake and would

add evidence of cyanide toxicity. Here the SvO2 is within normal limits (65-70).

13 MEDICAL

Questions

1. Responding to a small ER, you find a middle aged male patient presenting with altered mental status, hyperglycemia, and increased work of breathing. You note the following findings: HR 102, RR 32, SpO_2 99%, BP 142/85, blood sugar 300 mg/dL, and $EtCO_2$ of 65. Which of the following management options would best benefit the patient?

   A. Reduce the PEEP and the FiO_2
   B. Fluid bolus and insulin infusion
   C. Increased minute ventilation
   D. Sodium bicarbonate and calcium

2. You are transporting an adult DKA patient. Currently, they present with a blood glucose of 400 mg/dL, polyuria, BP of

132/76, RR 29, and EtCO2 of 44. Which of the following treatments is most appropriate?

A. Admin 40 mg of furosemide
B. Deliver 52 units of insulin
C. Provide 25 g of 50% dextrose
D. Give 1 L of isotonic crystalloid

3. You are investigating the history of a patient. Look at the medications below and choose the answer that suggests the patient has some form of depression on a TCA?

A. Midazolam hydrochloride
B. Buspirone hydrochloride
C. Fluoxetine hydrochloride
D. Nortriptyline hydrochloride

4. An older woman presents with severe weakness, hypotension, lower back pain, and vomiting. Her husband tells you that she has not taken her prednisone in several days because she has not been feeling well. Which of the following should you suspect?

A. Thyrotoxic crisis
B. Pheochromocytoma
C. Addisonian crisis
D. Cushing syndrome

5. After picking up an ARDS patient, you are formulating your plan on how to mechanically ventilate the patient.

Currently, their EtCO2 is 70 mmHg. You Decide to increase the minute ventilation to target a EtCO2 of 40. Which of the following set of findings would you most likely anticipate with this treatment?

A. Na+ drops 30 mEq/L & pH maintains
B. pH increases & K+ drops 1.5 mEq/L
C. pH increases & Phos falls by 4.1
D. Serum Ca+ increases by 2.7mEq/L

6. A patient with diabetic ketoacidosis would typically present with which of the following signs and/or symptoms?

A. Hypoglycemia and dehydration
B. Hyperglycemia and oliguria
C. Hypoglycemia and polyuria
D. Hyperglycemia and dehydration

7. Look at the following and identify the patient who is most at risk for hypothermia

A. 51-year-old man with coronary artery disease
B. 49-year-old man with hyperglycemia
C. 58-year-old woman with Cushing syndrome
D. 53-year-old woman with hypothyroidism

8. A 51-year-old male complains of generalized weakness that began about a 5 days ago. He is awake, alert with the

following vitals BP 142/77 mm Hg, pulse is 128 beats/min and irregular, and respirations are 18 breaths/min. The cardiac monitor reveals atrial fibrillation. The patient denies any significant medical problems and takes no medications. The most appropriate treatment would be which of the following?

A. Admin versed; perform cardioversion
B. Administer 0.25 mg/kg of diltiazem
C. 150 mg of amiodarone over 10 min
D. Vagal maneuvers; 6 mg of adenosine

9. A patient with a history of Grave's disease presents with anxiety, profuse sweating and a palpable goiter. Vitals are P 151, R 35 and labored, BP 84/42. Which working diagnosis is most likely?

A. Diabetes insipidus
B. Thyrotoxicosis
C. Cocaine toxicity
D. Myxedema

10. You are assessing a patient who presents with a melena and abdominal pain. Which of the following medical history findings is the most clinically significant?

A. Hypertension
B. von Willebrand disease
C. Type II diabetes mellitus
D. Hashimoto disease

11. You are called to a residence for a 39-year-old woman, who, according to her husband ate a casserole that had peanuts in it, which she is allergic to, and she currently has the following vitals: HR 102, RR 29, BP 72/50, SpO2 89%, and EtCO2 62. Which of the following is the most appropriate treatment?

    A. BVM with 8 of PEEP
    B. Intubate the patient
    C. Administer some epi
    D. Provide Benadryl to pt

12. A patient is being treated for acute adrenal insufficiency. Which of the following findings indicate the patient is responding favorably?

    A. decreasing serum sodium
    B. decreasing serum potassium
    C. decreasing blood glucose
    D. increasing urinary output

13. You are transporting a patient who presents with bruising (reportedly, they bruise easily recently), lymph node enlargement, and splenomegaly. These symptoms suggest which of the of the following?

    A. Leukemia
    B. Anemia
    C. Polycythemia
    D. Lymphoma

14. You are to transport a patient with esophageal varices. Which of the following would most suggest this pathophysiology?

    A. Hematemesis, jaundice, and hypertension
    B. Abdominal pain, headache, hyperkalemia
    C. High AST, hematochezia, severe polyuria
    D. Jaundice, hypotension, and head ache

15. You are called to transport a n adult patient from a rural ER. When reviewing the lab results from the clinic, you note that the patient's thyroid-stimulating hormone is 9.2 mcgU/mL (elevated). Which of the following conditions is consistent with this finding?

    A. Graves' disease
    B. Cushing syndrome
    C. An underactive thyroid
    D. Elevated T3/T4 levels

16. You are responding to a patient in anaphylactic shock. They currently present with BP 74/54, HR 108, severe uticaria, and wheezes. Which of the following is the most appropriate treatment for this condition?

    A. Epi: 0.3 to 0.5 mg IM
    B. 10cc/kg NS fluid bolus
    C. Surgical cricothyrotomy
    D. Benadryl 25-50 mg IV

17. Following prolonged dehydration, a 67-year-old man presents with hypotension, tachycardia, and oliguria. He has no past medical history. Which of the following is the MOST likely cause of his condition?

    A. Chronic renal failure
    B. Prerenal acute renal failure
    C. Postrenal acute renal failure
    D. Intrarenal acute renal failure

18. Your 60 y/o male patient presents with a pH 7.18, increased work of breathing, GCS of 14 (E4,V4,M6), and a blood sugar of 670 mg/dL. A 54 year old male presents with altered mental status and an increased work of breathing. The pH is reduced and the blood sugar is high. Which of the following conditions is the patient currently experiencing?

    A. (+) Graves' disease
    B. A mild form of HHNK
    C. Diabetic ketoacidosis
    D. (+) Hypothyroidism

19. Your adult complains of fatigue, malaise, constipation, and says she gets cold very fast. She reiterates that she cannot stand the cold. Which of the following medications would be most beneficial to the patient?

    A. Gram- antibiotics
    B. Gram+ antibiotics
    C. Dexamethasone
    D. Levothyroxine

20. Your assessment of a patient reveals a diffuse petechial rash. Which of the following hematologic disorders does this indicate?

    A. Hemolytic anemia
    B. Polycythemia vera
    C. Thrombocytopenia
    D. Leukopenia

Answers

---

1. (**C**) This patient presents and diabeticketo acidosis (hyper glycemia, fast respiratory rate, and altered mental status). It appears the patient is trying to breathe off the excess acid created by the DKA. In this case, the best solution is to increase the patient's minute ventilation during mechanical ventilation to help and assure enough acid is blown off. Reducing peep will only change the oxygenation effort; fluid and insulin may be warranted, but not a top priority; While sodium bicarb any beneficial, calcium is not war to this case therefore this answer selection is incorrect. The ultimate teaching point here is to not reduce the patient's compensatory respiratory effort. If you have only sedate in paralyzes patient and reduce their minute ventilation, the patient will get extremely acidotic. Always make sure you're watching your patient and making ventilator decisions based on end tidal CO2 and SpO2.

2. (**D**) Ultimately this patient needs fluids and some insulin (slow). The insulin dose here is too high no matter which type of insulin you gave. Lasix (furosemide is contraindicated in anyone with dehydration or hypovolemia. The fix for a high blood sugar isn't more blood sugar, so the D50 selection is out. Rehydrate the patient.

3. (**D**) Nortriptyline (Pamelor), amyltriptyline (Elavil), and clomipramine hydrochloride (Anafranil) are commonly prescribed tricyclic antidepressant (TCA) medications. Fluoxetine hydrochloride (Prozac) is a selective serotonin reuptake inhibitor (SSRI) that is also used to treat depression as well as obsessive-compulsive disorder. Midazolam hydrochloride (Versed) is a benzodiazepine sedative-hypnotic. Buspirone hydrochloride (Buspar) is an anxiolytic medication

4. (**C**) Signs and symptoms of acute adrenal insufficiency can manifest suddenly in what is called an Addisonian crisis. Abrupt cessation of corticosteroid therapy (i.e., prednisone, hydrocortisone) is the most common cause of an addisonian crisis. It may also be triggered by acute exacerbation of chronic adrenal insufficiency (Addison disease), usually brought on by stress, trauma, surgery, or a severe infection. In either case, cardiovascular collapse occurs due to a lack of the hormone cortisol; therefore, the chief clinical manifestation of an addisonian crisis is shock. Other signs and symptoms may include weakness; lethargy; fever; severe pain in the lower back, legs, or abdomen; and severe vomiting and diarrhea. Cushing syndrome is caused by excessive cortisol production by the

adrenal cortex; it may also occur if large amounts of corticosteroids are administered. Pheochromocytoma is an adrenal tumor that causes excessive release of epinephrine and norepinephrine; patients with this condition present with hypertension and tachycardia. Thyrotoxic crisis (thyroid storm) is a condition caused by critically high thyroid hormone levels, resulting in a hypermetabolic state. Signs and symptoms include severe tachycardia, hypertension, fever, altered mental status, and possibly heart failure.

5. (**B**) To answer this question you must have a working knowledge of the winter's formula, or ultimately that changing end tidal CO2 also changes the potassium in the same direction. Every 10 mmHg of change with EtCO2, the potassium will change by a factor of 0.5 in the same direction. Therefore if you were to change an EtCO2 by 25 mmHg, than you'd expect a change in potassium by 1.2 mEq/L, therefore the answer selection with this value is the correct answer.

6. (**D**) Diabetic ketoacidosis (DKA), also referred to as diabetic coma or hyperglycemic crisis, is characterized by hyperglycemia, polyuria (excessive urination), polydipsia (excessive thirst), and polyphagia (excessive hunger). Other findings include warm, dry skin, dehydration, and deep, rapid respirations (Kussmaul's respirations). The progression to DKA is typically slow, often over several hours to a few days. By contrast, insulin shock (hypoglycemic crisis) is characterized by a rapid onset, often within a few minutes.

7. (**D**) Hypothyroidism is a condition in which the thyroid gland produces too little T3 (triiodothyronine) and T4 (thyroxine), resulting in a decrease in the metabolic rate. Any time the metabolic rate decreases, heat energy production is reduced; therefore, the patient is prone to hypothermia. Cushing syndrome is caused by excessive cortisol production by the adrenal glands or by excessive use of cortisol or other similar glucocorticoid hormones (i.e., prednisone, hydrocortisone, methylprednisolone). This increase in cortisol would cause an increase in the metabolic rate. Patient's with Cushing syndrome are not at risk for hypothermia, nor are patients with hyperglycemia or coronary artery disease.

8. (**B**) This patient should not be cardioverted because it has potentially been longer than 48 hours from onset, meaning if you cardiovert, and emboli could be thrown from their stagnant right atrium to the lungs causing a PE. This patient is hemodynamically stable and is not in need of electrical therapy. Appropriate treatment for a patient with A-Fib or atrial flutter (A-Flutter) with a rapid ventricular rate (RVR) involves controlling the ventricular rate with a calcium-channel blocker. Diltiazem (Cardizem) is the most common medicine used for this condition. Vagal maneuvers and adenosine are for narrow complex (ventricular) tachycardias.

9. (**B**) Thyrotoxicosis refers to the presence of too much thyroid hormone in the body and hyperthyroidism is when thyrotoxicosis is due to overproduction of thyroid hormone by the thyroid gland. The goiter, sweating, and anxiety all point to hyperthyroidism, therefore,

thyrotoxicosis is the best answer. Grave's disease is the most common cause of hyperthyroidism. Myxedema is a term used synonymously with severe hypothyroidism. DI is a disorder of salt and water metabolism marked by intense thirst and heavy urination.

10. (**B**) The presence of von Willebrand disease in a patient with internal or external bleeding should concern you the most. Von Willebrand disease, a bleeding disorder similar to hemophilia, is caused by a deficiency of von Willebrand factor (vWF), a blood clotting protein. vWF circulates attached to factor VIII, another blood clotting protein. As a consequence of von Willebrand disease, the normal process of hemostasis is interrupted and the patient will continue to bleed. Hashimoto disease, also called Hashimoto thyroiditis, is a cause of hyperthyroidism; it is an autoimmune disorder that affects the thyroid-stimulating hormone (TSH) receptors. While hypertension, Hashimoto disease, and type II diabetes can certainly complicate the clinical picture of any sick or injured patient, bleeding disorders in a patient with active bleeding would clearly be the most detrimental.

11. (**C**) This patient is experiencing severe anaphylaxis. Since blood pressure has been affected (a sign of severe anaphylaxis) epi is needed to increase BP. Additionally, it will combat tissue edema, increase airway size, and reduce the histamine effect.

12. (**B**) Clinical manifestations of Addison's disease include hyperkalemia and a decrease in potassium level indicates improvement. Decreasing serum sodium and decreasing blood glucose indicate that treatment has not been

effective. Changes in urinary output are not an effective way of monitoring treatment for Addison's disease.

13. (**A**) Leukemia is cancer of the blood, and is caused by an abnormal proliferation (production by multiplication) of leukocytes (white blood cells) in the bone marrow. Leukemic cells impair the normal production of red blood cells (RBCs), white blood cells (WBCs), and platelets (thrombocytes); this results in anemia, leukopenia (low WBC count), and easy bleeding due to thrombocytopenia (low platelet count). In leukemia, excessive white blood cells accumulate in major organs (i.e., spleen, liver, brain, and lymph), causing them to become enlarged (i.e., splenomegaly [enlarged spleen], adenopathy [enlarged lymph nodes], hepatomegaly [enlarged liver]). Other signs and symptoms of leukemia include bone pain (due to increased pressure in the medullary canal of the bone), fever, fatigue, night sweats, and weight loss.

14. (**A**) The jaundice gives away that the patient has a liver pathophysiology, and the throwing up blood in the face of liver pathology strongly suggests esophageal varices. The other three answer selections are forms of GI bleeds, but the jaundice is telltale in this case.

15. (**C**) Hypothyroidism is a condition in which the thyroid gland produces too little T3 (triiodothyronine) and T4 (thyroxine), resulting in a decrease in the metabolic rate. Any time the metabolic rate decreases, heat energy production is reduced; therefore, the patient is prone to hypothermia. Cushing syndrome is caused by excessive cortisol production by the adrenal glands or by excessive use of cortisol or other similar glucocorticoid hormones

(i.e., prednisone, hydrocortisone, methylprednisolone). This increase in cortisol would cause an increase in the metabolic rate. Patient's with Cushing syndrome are not at risk for hypothermia, nor are patients with hyperglycemia or coronary artery disease.

16. (**A**) This patient is experiencing severe anaphylaxis. Since blood pressure has been affected (a sign of severe anaphylaxis) epi is needed to increase BP. Additionally, it will combat tissue edema, increase airway size, and reduce the histamine effect.

17. (**B**) Acute renal failure (ARF) is a sudden decrease in glomerular filtration rate (GFR), which causes toxins to accumulate in the blood. ARF is classified into three types, based on the area in which the failure occurs: prerenal, intrarenal, and postrenal. Prerenal ARF is caused by hypoperfusion of the kidneys; not enough blood passes into the glomeruli for them to produce filtrate. The most common causes of prerenal ARF are hypovolemia (blood loss or severe dehydration), trauma, sepsis, shock, and heart failure. Intrarenal ARF involves damage to one of three areas in the kidney: the glomeruli capillaries and small blood vessels, the cells of the renal tubules, or the renal parenchyma. This type of ARF can be caused by immune-mediated diseases (i.e., type I diabetes) or by certain medications. Postrenal ARF is caused by obstruction of urine flow from the kidneys. The source of this obstruction is often a blockage of the urethra by an enlarged prostate gland, renal calculi (kidney stones), or strictures. As a result, pressure in the nephrons is increased, which causes them to stop functioning. Chronic

renal failure is progressive and irreversible inadequate kidney function caused by the permanent loss of nephrons. This disease develops over months or years. More than half of all cases are caused by systemic disease, such as hypertension or diabetes.

18. (**C**) This presentation (acidosis, hyperglycemia, and tachypnea) all lead toward the diagnosis of diabetic ketoacidosis, or DKA. Remember, the biggest difference between DKA and HHNK is the fact that HHNK produces just enough insulin to prevent the cells from having to undergo anaerobic metabolism, and thus prevent acidosis.

19. (**D**) This patient is experiencing hypothyroidism: condition of hyposecretion of the thyroid gland causing low thyroid levels in the blood that result in sluggishness, slow pulse, and often obesity. It is treated with Synthroid or Levothyroxine. When these patients will continue to remain sluggish, slow and cold intolerant without this medication.

20. (**C**) Of the conditions listed, only one would cause a petechial rash. Thrombocytopenia, a reduction in the number of circulating platelets, can cause cutaneous bleeding and bleeding from the mucous membranes (i.e., nosebleeds, rectal bleeding). Petechiae, tiny purple or red spots that appear on the skin, is caused by bleeding within the skin or under the mucous membranes. Localized petichiae may be harmless; however, a diffuse petechial rash indicates significant thrombocytopenia. Leukopenia is a reduction in the number of white blood cells (leukocytes); this condition places the patient at increased risk for infection. Polycythemia vera, also called primary

polycythemia, is a hematologic disorder in which the bone marrow makes too many red blood cells; it may also result in an overproduction of white blood cells and platelets. Hemolytic anemia is a form of anemia caused by hemolysis, the abnormal breakdown (lysis) of red blood cells.

14 ENVIRONMENTAL

Questions

1. You arrive to find your patient in a cold environment and the patient is having trouble answering questions and is slurring their words. If this is related to temperature, then what is the patient's current temperature?

   A. 32-35°C
   B. 30-31°C
   C. 28-30°C
   D. 25-28°C

2. A patient in your care is experiencing hypothermia from prolonged extrication in February. As you are loading them into the aircraft they are nearly dropped and impacted the stretcher with high force. The patient entered a ventricular

fibrillation rhythm. What would you assess the patient's current temperature to be?

A. < 90° F
B. 91-93° F
C. 95-97° F
D. > 97° F

3. Severe hypothermia is recognized as a body temperature below what temperature (in degrees Celsius).

A. 34°
B. 30°
C. 26°
D. 22°

4. Your patient is a hiker who got caught in a snow storm. They were discovered with frostbitten feet and hands. As you approach the patient in the ER, you note the patient is lying down on the bed, the family is rubbing his hands to keep them warm, and the patient has pushed off the blanket from covering him. Which of the following is the most appropriate response to this situation?

A. Replace the blanket to cover patient
B. Receive report and transport patient
C. Ask family to stop rubbing hands
D. Have the family sit up the patient

5. A patient was rescued from flood waters. They were trapped on the roof of their car for hours. Once in the

rescue aircraft, you notice that they stop shivering. You recall this is the temperature that shivering stops.

A. 95° F
B. 91° F
C. 83° F
D. 89° F

6. A football player experiences heat stroke in the middle of two a day practices in August. What would be your most likely finding?

A. Hyponatremia
B. Hyperglycemia
C. Hypokalemia
D. Hypercalcemia

7. Your hypothermic patient was found behind an abandoned store without a pulse. There is no dependent lividity or rigor mortis yet. Which of the following is the most appropriate action?

A. Support ventilations and withhold CPR
B. Call the time of death and the coroner
C. Begin CPR and attempt to rewarm patient
D. Begin CPR immediately and transport

8. A football player becomes delirious, stops sweating, and is removed from play. You are transporting him now and he presents with nausea, 102° F, dry skin, and dark colored

urine. Which of the following is the most appropriate treatment for this patient?

A. Aggressive fluid therapy
B. Administer glycogen
C. Monitor oxygen saturation
D. Administer H2 blockers

9. You confirm that your hypothermic patient is in cardiac arrest. At what temperature (in degrees F) can you begin administering medications?

A. 86
B. 82
C. 90
D. 93

10. Your patient is a homeless person who had been found outside in the cold and unconscious. He responds to only painful stimuli and is very cold to the touch. The patient presents with the following: HR 50, BP 80/40, and RR 6. Which of the following is the most appropriate management for this patient?

A. Active rewarming
B. Assist ventilations
C. Apply ECG monitor
D. Intubate the patient

Answers

1. (**A**) At 32-35 degrees, the patient is experiencing the "umbles" which include the fumbles, stumbles, mumbles, and crumbles. This indicates severe hypothermia. This is simply a memorization question. You'll need to know the various temperatures that relate to physiological changes in your environmental emergency patient.

2. (**A**) Patient's below 90° F are pre-disposed to ventricular fibrillation should the body be handled roughly during the transition of the patient from the scene into the aircraft or transport vehicle. At 82.4°F, the heart can spontaneously enter ventricular fibrillation. Make sure to handle extremely cold patients gently.

3. (**B**) This is simply a memorization question. You'll need to know the various temperatures that relate to physiological changes in your environmental emergency patient. Additionally, know how to convert F° to C°: to convert temperatures in degrees Fahrenheit to Celsius, subtract 32 and multiply by .5556 (or 5/9).

4. (**C**) You should never rub frozen parts. Ice crystals form in the frostbitten tissues. Rubbing a frostbitten area will move the ice crystals in the tissues, causing trauma and worsening the injury.

5. (B) As a patient's body temperature continues to drop, once they reach 91° F, shivering stops. Commit this temperature and concept to memory.

6. (**A**) A key piece of information here is the fact that this is a football player practicing twice a day in August. Football players drink a lot of fluids, a lot of hypotonic fluids (water), which can stimulate hyponatremia. Additionally, player sweat a lot of sodium out, therefore with these two pieces of information, the most likely find it would be hyponatremia. The liver will usually release glucose and lower glucose states, unless the liver is damaged. It is safe to assume that this patient you most likely has a healthy liver. Hyperkalemia is and heat stroke, however the answer selection and this question his hypokalemia, therefore it is an incorrect answer selection. Hypocalcemia Typically occurs because debits muscle will bind more calcium, however in this case, the answer selection is "hypercalcemia" therefore it is an incorrect answer selection.

7. (**D**) You should begin CPR immediately and transport the patient. After a patient has been submersed in cold water, the effects of hypothermia and the mammalian diving reflex will increase the time during which the patient could be successfully resuscitated. Rewarming severely hypothermic patients must begin from the core and work outward to prevent lactic acid wash out. Once vasoconstriction in the periphery is relieved from rewarming, the periphery opens up the dump's all of the previously sequestered lactic acid into systemic circulation causing near-immediate acidosis. Therefore, the answer to this question involves be giving CPR immediately WITHOUT rewarming the patient.

8. (**C**) Ultimately, myoglobinuria should be treated with lots of fluids to help clear out the kidney of myoglobin and prevent blockage within the kidney itself.

9. (**A**) This is simply a memorization question. You'll need to know the various temperatures that relate to physiological changes in your environmental emergency patient.

10. (**B**) The best answer in this case is to assist ventilations. Even though we do not know the exact temp, cold to touch with depressed vital signs indicates an advanced hypothermic state. Anytime all vitals drop because of hypothermia, it has to be an advanced progression of the pathophysiology. When patients are this cold, then active re-warming is contraindicated until the patients are warmed passively. Rewarming too early will cause a reduction of peripheral vasoconstriction and releasing lots of lactic acid into central circulation.

ABOUT THE AUTHOR

Charlie Swearingen first conceived the dream of becoming a flight clinician while he was still in paramedic school. He decided that instead of blithely waiting for a position to become available, he would begin arming himself with the professional achievements that would eventually earn him a spot on a revered, level 1 helicopter in Mississippi. He is in the middle of a PhD in physiology, is an educator for the world's largest air medical service provider, and also is a world class athlete on the US National Men's Sitting volleyball team. He eventually founded Meducation Specialists, a company dedicated to developing and deploying world-class medical education.

Made in the USA
Columbia, SC
22 December 2022